By David Zinczenko

Eat This, Not That! The No-Diet Weight-Loss Solution

Eat This, Not That! For Kids

Eat This, Not That! Supermarket Survival Guide

Eat This, Not That! Restaurant Survival Guide

Eat This, Not That! Best (& Worst) Foods in America!

Cook This, Not That! Kitchen Survival Guide

Cook This, Not That! Skinny Comfort Food

Cook This, Not That! Easy & Awesome 350-Calorie Meals

Grill This, Not That! Backyard Survival Guide

Drink This, Not That! The No-Diet Weight-Loss Solution

Eat This, Not That! No-Diet Diet

The 8-Hour Diet

The New Abs Diet

The New Abs Diet for Women

The New Abs Diet Cookbook

The Abs Diet Eat Right Every Time Guide

The Abs Diet Ultimate Nutrition Handbook

The Abs Diet 6-Minute Meals for 6-Pack Abs

Men, Love & Sex: The Complete User's Guide for Women

Eat It to Beat It!

Eat This, Not That! When You're Expecting
(co-authored with Dr. Jennifer Ashton)

Zero Belly Diet

Zero Belly Cookbook

Zero Belly Smoothies

ZERO
SUGAR
DIET

ZERO SUGAR DIET

The 14-Day Plan to Flatten
Your Belly, Crush Cravings, and
Help Keep You Lean for Life

DAVID ZINCZENKO

with Stephen Perrine

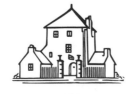

Ballantine Books
New York

Copyright © 2016 by David Zinczenko

Published in the United States by Ballantine Books, an imprint of Random House, a division of Penguin Random House LLC, New York.

BALLANTINE and the HOUSE colophon are registered trademarks of Penguin Random House LLC.

ISBN 978-0-345-54798-9
Ebook ISBN 978-0-345-54800-9

Photographs by George Karabotos

Printed in the United States of America on acid-free paper

randomhousebooks.com

2 4 6 8 9 7 5 3 1

First Edition

Book design by Joe Heroun

For every American who's struggled with their weight. Today you take back control.

CONTENTS

Introduction

IMAGINE FOR A MOMENT that scientists discovered a new, virulent virus. This virus caused chronic, unrelenting, irreversible obesity, and sufferers often went on to experience heart failure and liver damage, as well as blindness, arthritis, gout, and even cancer. Imagine, too, that the first symptoms of infection were fatigue and abdominal weight gain. You'd be pretty worried if you noticed your belly expanding and your energy waning, wouldn't you?

Imagine that to diagnose this virus, doctors gave you a simple blood test that looked for elevated blood glucose, elevated blood pressure, and high cholesterol. And that, once diagnosed, the virus was completely treatable, as long as you caught it in time.

Now imagine that doctors were being incentivized by big business and the government not to tell you that this virus exists, and not to recommend the simple cure—and, in fact, they go one step further, shaping dietary recommendations that cause the disease to spread. And as a result, one in three Americans was already infected, and on his or her way to dying from the disease.

If that seems far-fetched, it's not. In fact, it's pretty much what's happening today, with one small difference: It's not a virus that doctors are keeping quiet about. It's sugar.

The Zero Sugar Diet is the cure.

By following this simple fourteen-day plan, you will quickly and efficiently bring your body into perfect balance, and begin dropping excess pounds at a rapid pace. And in doing so, you'll discover a new way of walking through the world, one that keeps you safely out of the grasp of weight gain and one of the biggest diseases of our time. And you'll do it by eating foods you love—yes, even foods from your favorite restaurants and supermarkets; even burgers, bacon, and pasta. You will flatten your belly, improve your health, and look, feel, and live better than ever. And you will set yourself up for a lifetime of effortless success.

Zero Sugar Diet works because it targets the most virulent virus of all: added sugars. And it was developed with the cutting-edge recommendations of the world's more preeminent medical associations in mind.

Earlier this year, the Food and Drug Administration announced approval of a new Nutrition Facts label, which includes a separate line for added sugars, forcing companies to list what's added and what's natural for the first time. And the U.S. Department of Agriculture, the World Health Organization, and the American Heart Association have all come out vociferously against added sugar: The AHA recommends no more than 100 calories per day from added sugars, or six teaspoons, for women, and 150 calories (nine teaspoons) for men.

And those recommendations make complete sense: New research suggests that for every 5 percent of total calories you consume from added sweeteners, your risk of diabetes increases by 18 percent. That means for the average woman, who consumes about 1,858 calories a day, all you need to eat is 93 calories a day of added sugar to significantly boost your risk. There are 4 calories in a gram of sugar, so that means about 23 grams of added sugar per day will put you directly in the path of an oncoming diabetes train.

And you don't have to live on Jolly Ranchers to reach that number. Here are some seemingly healthy foods that put you over your daily limit with just one serving:

Dannon Fruit on the Bottom Cherry Yogurt: **24 grams**
Quaker Natural Granola Oats & Honey: **26 grams**

PowerBar Performance Energy Vanilla Crisp: **26 grams**
Tazo Organic Iced Green Tea: **30 grams**
Ocean Spray Cran-Apple: **31 grams**

The problem is, even if you're vigilant, even if you read the labels and make it a rule not to eat anything with more than 10 grams of added sugar, the numbers add up, because sugar is in everything—especially foods it doesn't belong in, like bread, peanut butter, pasta sauce, salad dressing, and oatmeal. In the form of high-fructose corn syrup (HFCS), it even coats the outside of your Advil caplets!

Here's how easily your numbers can add up: Start your day with Quaker Instant Apple and Cinnamon Oatmeal (9 grams of sugar per serving), have a peanut butter sandwich for lunch with Jif (3 grams) on Pepperidge Farm Whole Wheat Farmhouse Bread (another 3 grams per slice), and then enjoy a dinner of pasta with Ragu Old-World Style Sauce (6 grams of added sugars—it's the third ingredient after tomato paste and soybean oil). A simple salad with Kraft Zesty Lime Vinaigrette adds another 3 grams. No cookies, no ice cream, no cake, no soda, not even a single bite of chocolate, but you've consumed 27 grams of added sugars, or 6.75 teaspoons' worth—more than what a woman should eat in an entire day.

Doesn't that piss you off—especially when none of those foods actually requires added sugar? It's the reason why, on average, we now get twenty-two teaspoons per day—88 grams of added sugar, or about four times our safety limit! It's not just because we're chowing down on too many Little Debbies. It's because our healthy foods, like salads, oatmeal, and peanut butter, are being spiked with the same poison.

Of course, your doctor has already gone over all of this with you, so . . .

Oh wait, she hasn't? How can that be? Virulent epidemic + medical consensus + simple remedy ought to lead to an easy, universal cure.

DECODING THE NEW NUTRITION LABEL

Old   **New**

Nutrition Facts

Serving Size 2/3 cup (55g)
Servings Per Container About 8

Amount Per Serving

Calories 230	Calories from Fat 72
	% Daily Value*
Total Fat 8g	**12%**
Saturated Fat 1g	**5%**
Trans Fat 0g	
Cholesterol 0mg	**0%**
Sodium 160mg	**7%**
Total Carbohydrate 37g	**12%**
Dietary Fiber 4g	**16%**
Sugars 1g	
Protein 3g	
Vitamin A	10%
Vitamin C	8%
Calcium	20%
Iron	45%

* Percent Daily Values are based on a 2,000 calorie diet.
Your daily value may be higher or lower depending on
your calorie needs.

	Calories:	2,000	2,500
Total Fat	Less than	65g	80g
Sat Fat	Less than	20g	25g
Cholesterol	Less than	300mg	300mg
Sodium	Less than	2,400mg	2,400mg
Total Carbohydrate		300g	375g
Dietary Fiber		25g	30g

Nutrition Facts

8 servings per container
Serving size 2/3 cup (55g)

Amount per serving
Calories 230

	% Daily Value*
Total Fat 8g	**10%**
Saturated Fat 1g	**5%**
Trans Fat 0g	
Cholesterol 0mg	**0%**
Sodium 160mg	**7%**
Total Carbohydrate 37g	**13%**
Dietary Fiber 4g	**14%**
Total Sugars 12g	
Includes 10g Added Sugars	**20%**
Protein 3g	
Vitamin D 2mcg	10%
Calcium 260mg	20%
Iron 8mg	45%
Potassium 235mg	6%

* The % Daily Value (DV) tells you how much a nutrient in
a serving of food contributes to a daily diet. 2,000 calories
a day is used for general nutrition advice.

The **serving size** is bigger and bolder, so you can't miss it. When it was smaller, sneaky food manufacturers could more easily define their "servings" as tiny, making their overall nutrition look healthier.

The **calorie count** will now be bigger, so you'll keep that top of mind.

This is the biggest change, and the most revolutionary: Now you'll know which sugars come from natural sources, and which are added. On *Zero Sugar Diet*, you want this number to be zero.

But there's a reason why you haven't heard about this issue from your doctor. That's why I had to write this book. The reason starts exactly 50 years ago, fueled by a conspiracy unveiled only just this year.

How the Sugar Industry Dug Us into a Hole

Open your mouth and take a look back there at your teeth. See any fillings? If so, you may consider cavities a normal part of growing up. But maybe you shouldn't.

Back in 1966, President Lyndon Johnson wanted, as he put it, a "national attack on disease and disability." To launch it, he asked all of the directors of the various National Institutes of Health to submit documents showing that they had one or more diseases in their sights.

Now, if you're the director of the National Cancer Institute or the National Heart, Lung and Blood Institute, you've got plenty of diseases to go after. But what if you're the director of the National Institute of Dental Research (NIDR)? You've pretty much got just one boogeyman to chase, and so the NIDR announced a targeted research initiative called the National Caries Program, with the goal of eliminating cavities in children within ten years.

Imagine that: The U.S. government believed it could eliminate all cavities in children—100 percent clean checkups—by the time Reese Witherspoon was born!

The driving force behind this promise: Recent research that found that sucrose—table sugar—caused bacteria to adhere to teeth, causing decay. A combination of fluoridation, research into the bacteria itself, and, most significantly, dietary modifications to reduce sugar consumption would end the plague of cavities within a decade, the NIDR's director claimed.

As *Mad Men*'s Don Draper advised, "If you don't like what's being said, change the conversation." And the sugar industry most definitely did not like what was being said. So they began funding research that would divert attention away from the notion that reducing sugar intake was crucial to preventing cavities. The International Sugar Research Foundation (ISRF)—a precursor to today's Sugar Association—began funding research into cavities, trying to push researchers away from the idea of reducing sugar intake and focusing instead on finding a vaccine against the disease, according to documents summarized in a 2015 report in the journal *PLOS Medicine*. The ISRF orchestrated a massive outreach to leading scientists, eventually setting up its own task force. By the time the first NIDR Caries Task Force Steering Committee was established in 1969, only one of the nine committee members wasn't already affiliated with the ISRF. And by the time the National Caries Program was launched in 1971, the idea of reducing sugar intake was pretty much pooh-poohed; about 40 percent of the NCP's report was taken verbatim or closely paraphrased from the ISRF.

And that's why you grew up with cavities.

Meanwhile, in a stunning new discovery uncovered just this year, internal sugar industry documents suggest that researchers—including ones from Harvard—were paid by the sugar industry under the table to publish studies that minimized the link between sugar and heart disease, pointing the finger instead at saturated fat. This resulted in years of dietary guidelines based on misinformation. "They were able to derail the discussion about sugar for decades," Stanton Glantz, an author of the *JAMA Internal Medicine* paper, told *The New York Times*.

Poisoning the Well

Today, the sugar and soda industries are doing very much the same thing with another disease, obesity. Thanks in part to the lobbying of the food industry, sugar consumption rose by 25 percent between 1970 and 2000, in almost exact parallel with the increase in high-fructose corn syrup production and obesity, according to a review by the Union of Concerned Scientists. The organization identified five separate tactics used by the food industry to help keep the sugar flowing: attacking the science linking sugar and obesity; hiring scientists to work on behalf of the industry; influencing academia through funding; undermining federal, state, and local policy through lobbying and PR campaigns; and spreading misinformation to the public.

For a solid example of that last point, you can check out the website for the Global Energy Balance Network, which seeks to "be the voice of science in ending obesity." Its premise is eating more calories—of any kind—and exercising more is the best way to maintain a healthy weight. In other words, if you're fat, it's because you don't exercise enough, not because of the quality or quantity of the food you're eating. Which is a good message to get out there if you're a company that sells high-calorie, nutrition-free foods and beverages.

So it won't surprise you to learn that the Global Energy Balance Network is owned by Coca-Cola—although you won't see that fact listed anywhere on the site.

In fact, since the USDA, the AHA, and the WHO all issued their warnings against sugar in 2014, many scientists have begun to worry that the sugar industry and its supporters, like soda and candy manufacturers, seem poised to pull another scientific-looking rabbit out of their hats, like they did back in 1966.

Their worries seem well-founded. Coca-Cola was recently unmasked as the number one sponsor of the Academy of Pediatrics' HealthyChildren.org website, and it has given nearly $3 million to the academy over the past six years, according to *The New York Times*. Other beneficiaries of the company's largesse: the American College of Cardiology ($3.1 million), the American Academy of Family Physicians ($3.5 million), the American Cancer Society ($2 million), and the Academy of Nutrition and Dietetics ($1.7 million). And recent studies finding that a lack of energy expenditure in adolescents contributed greatly to the obesity crisis turn out to have been funded by Coke.

In a 2013 review of literature in *PLOS Medicine*, the authors looked at eighteen scientific conclusions drawn from systematic reviews of studies on the link between sugar-sweetened beverage consumption and weight gain or obesity. Among reviews conducted by scientists without any reported conflict of interest, ten out of twelve found that sodas and other sugary beverages could be a risk factor for weight gain. But among studies that were funded by the food industry, five out of six found exactly the opposite. What a coincidence!

In explaining the company's position, Sandy Douglas, the president of Coca-Cola North America, told *The New York Times*, "I suspect that completely eliminating [sodas] is not necessary for kids to be healthy any more than eliminating ice cream, birthday cake or cookies."

But the fact is, eliminating that one single can of Coke *is* necessary. It contains 39 grams of added sugar; sugar makes up 100 percent of its 140 calories. A 2009 study at UCLA found that adults who drank one sugary beverage per day were 27 percent more likely to be classified as overweight than those who drank less. Just one daily Coke means you're consuming an additional thirty-nine pounds of sugar a year. In fact, scientists writing in the journal *Circulation* in 2015 estimated that eliminating sugar-sweetened beverages could save 184,000 lives a year—133,000 from diabetes, 45,000 from heart disease, and 6,450 from cancer.

But while it may take quite a bit of tap dancing for the junk food industry to convince us that sugar doesn't make us fat or sick (or, for that matter, give us cavities), it's easy for the business interests to keep us just a little bit confused.

For example, consider food labels. As you've probably sussed out by now, ingredients are listed on the labels in a particular order, according to how much of the product is made up of those individual ingredients. That's why food companies, fully aware that we know what they're up to, have started to list individual compounds under less scary sounding names. For example, when you see that the first four ingredients listed on the label of a PowerBar Vanilla Crisp Performance Bar are cane invert syrup, maltodextrin, fructose, and dextrose, what you might not quite grasp is that all four are forms of sugar. (Also listed later on in the ingredients list: sugar.)

That's why nutrition labels are tricky. Manufacturers would prefer to add five different types of sugar, and list them individually, than to use just a single source of sweetness and have it be ingredient number one on their label. So you'll often see things like molasses, coconut nectar, corn syrup, barley malt, and more listed, when they all add up to the same thing: a sugar rush. Even more confusing, some foods like yogurts have a certain amount of naturally occurring sugars, which are found in all dairy products, and then added sugars, which are added by manufacturers to turn our taste buds into seven-year-olds again. And remember, it's the added sugars, specifically, that health organizations want you to be concerned about.

To help you understand what you're eating better, the Food and Drug Administration proposed a simple change: Make the calorie count on the label larger, and add a new line under total sugars that told you how much of the sugar you were eating was "added sugar."

The reaction of the sugar industry? They started buzzing like a toddler who just pounded a Mountain Dew Big Gulp.

In fact, the proposal drew criticisms from the expected sources—the Sugar Association, the American Bakers Association, the Corn Refiners Association, and Nestlé—but also from places you wouldn't expect. For example, cranberry farmers are up in arms because manufacturers add sugar to most cranberry-based products to make them less bitter. And the sugar industry continues to battle against it. In a 2015 letter to the USDA, Sugar Association president Andrew C. Briscoe III argued, "There is not a preponderance of scientific evidence [linking] 'added sugars' intake to serious disease or negative health outcomes."

Including, his letter said, cavities.

Zero Sugar Diet is my response to him. But it's dedicated to you. Whether you want to change your body, improve your health or looks, or live longer and feel younger, in fourteen days, you'll be stronger, sexier, and better than ever—finally free from added sugar.

THE ZERO SUGAR

You'll enjoy three filling meals and one delicious snack per day.
Just make sure every serving includes:

► **A ZERO SUGAR CARB**

Vegetables (fresh or frozen)

Whole Fruit (fresh or frozen)

Beans/legumes

Unsweetened whole grains and cereals
(brown rice, quinoa, oats)

or Nuts/seeds

Plenty of fiber and no added sugar here! Eat them until you're satisfied.

► **A POWER PROTEIN**

Eggs, fish, Greek yogurt, or lean meat
(turkey, chicken, lean beef, roast pork)

These will keep your belly full and build fat-burning muscle fast.

► **A HEALTHY DRINK**

Water, tea, milk, or even wine in moderation

No juice—ever—or any beverage with added sugars. And limit alcohol to one glass of wine a day, namely the low-sugar varieties listed in the back of this book.

DIET AT-A-GLANCE

▶ **EXERCISE** (Optional)

To turbocharge your weight loss, I've developed a series of Sugar Burner Workouts you can do at home or in the gym—quickly and easily!

AND FOR PACKAGED GOODS, FIND A NATURAL AND SATISFYING SWEET SPOT

Want to add a canned soup? Buy a pasta? Choose a spaghetti sauce? Pick a protein bar? During the first fourteen days of *Zero Sugar Diet*, whenever you buy a food that comes packaged, simply read the label. If it has any added sugars, toss it. Then after the first fourteen days, if it has more sugar than fiber, it's not for you. Everything else is in the Sweet Spot and is good to go.

AND WE MADE IT EASY!

Too busy to check every label for yourself? No worries—we did it for you! Just choose any of the 600 popular supermarket foods listed in this book—or via our newsletter at **thezerosugardiet.com**—or cook up any of our fifty easy-to-make breakfast, lunch, dinner, and snack recipes. All are low in added sugar, high in fiber, and satisfyingly delicious.

SO THERE YOU ARE:

Just four simple guidelines. Follow them and you're guaranteed to have more energy, feel better than ever, and shed fat fast. Our test panelists lost up to sixteen pounds in just two weeks!

chapter 1

STRIP AWAY SUGAR, STRIP AWAY TROUBLE

FOURTEEN DAYS.

That's all it will take to change your body. So, it's no wonder that when I announced a test program for *Zero Sugar Diet*, more than eleven hundred signed up in twenty-four hours. As soon as the word went out among the five million people who visit EatThis.com every month, we began hearing from fans who were trying to control their sugar addictions but struggling each and every day.

Our test panelists not only lived *Zero Sugar Diet*, but they documented—on a day-by-day basis—the remarkable changes that happened within their own bodies. Energy levels soared. Waistlines shrank. Blood pressure and cholesterol numbers plummeted. Muscles became toned and lean.

This unique day-by-day approach will help to keep you motivated as you compare yourself with, and even exceed, the success of the test panelists, many of whom struggled with real sugar addictions. When you reduce your sugar intake using this program, while slowing its impact on your body, a number of amazing things will happen, with shocking rapidity:

1. You'll Start Burning Fat

Immediately. Reducing your intake of calorie-dense sugar carbs automatically reduces the amount of calories you're consuming on a daily basis, which forces your body to burn fat stored around your midsection for energy, rather than the sugars it takes from carbohydrates.

2. You'll Feel Less Hungry

As your body detects that you've started to lose weight, your hunger hormones get furious. They start firing off signals to your brain telling you that winter's approaching, the barbarian hordes are at the gate, and you'd better consume every calorie in sight in order to prepare for the famine ahead.

This plan uses the power of fiber to counteract that basic instinct. By slowing the progress of carbohydrates through your body, fiber helps give you a continuous, steady dose of energy, so you never get the "I'm empty" signal. Oh, you'll eat plenty of food, but not because you're ravenous. Because it tastes so good!

3. Your Belly Will Get Flatter

One of the first things you notice when you replace simple carbs with high-fiber foods is that your belly begins to flatten out—literally within days. The reason: Most Americans only take in 15 of the recommended 25 to 38 grams per day, according to the Institute of Medicine. As a result, the healthy gut microbes that keep us lean have less to munch on, and the unhealthy microbes—which feast on sugar—take over. Those are the little buggers that cause bloating and make your belly look bigger than it actually is. In fact, an increase in the "bad" belly biome bacteria—a family called Firmicutes—is one of the most noticeable differences between Americans in the lean 1980s and those in the fat 2000s. I'll show you how this plan changes the way your gut acts and feels, and why fourteen days is all it takes to shrink your waist size by as much as seven inches.

4. You'll Slash Your Risk of Diabetes

Eating too many simple sugars can wreak havoc in your body in both the short and long term. The more of these quickly digested carbs you consume, the more insulin your pancreas produces, eventually leading to insulin resistance and possibly type 2 diabetes.

5. Your Muscles Will Get Stronger

In one of the most stunning studies of recent years, scientists have linked refined sugar to a condition called sarcopenia—basically, age-related loss of muscle mass. It happens because added sugar actually blocks the body's ability to synthesize protein into muscle. (Spending big bucks on protein supplements? If they have added sugar, they're probably hurting, not enhancing, your ability to build lean muscle.) By reducing the impact of sugar, this plan will keep your muscles younger and stronger—protecting you from injury and helping you to burn fat faster and more efficiently.

6. You'll Feel More Energized

By slowing your body's absorption of carbohydrates, you'll keep your body and your brain more fully fueled all the time, beating both general physical fatigue and the brain fog that can often accompany it. You'll no longer need to make poor food choices as a way of getting quick energy, and you won't be dragging through those afternoon hours.

Raising (Sugar) Cain

You can see why I had to write this book.

In fact, for the past two decades, I have been investigating the secrets of the food industry. And I've gotten tired of marketers trying to blame us, the American people, for the obesity crisis. In 2002, I published a controversial *New York Times* op-ed in defense of a group of kids who were suing McDonald's for making them fat.

A lot of people thought I was nuts: Suing McDonald's for making you fat is like suing Porsche for making you get a speeding ticket. But at least that Porsche comes with a speedometer. Fifteen years ago the idea of there being calorie counts and nutrition information for restaurant food was unheard of. There was absolutely no way of knowing how many calories were in that Big Mac. And, as I pointed out, if you drive down any highway in America, it's a lot easier to find a set of golden arches than it is a place to buy a grapefruit.

That op-ed was the opening salvo in what has become a career-long crusade. When I wrote *The Abs Diet* in 2004, I dedicated it to "every American who has taken up arms in the battle against obesity." I explained why counting calories while you diet and exercise wasn't the way to lose weight: Simply put, it takes far too long to burn off 300 calories, and no time at all to eat them back up. Instead, I focused on quality nutrition and the importance of boosting metabolism—long before "boost your metabolism" became a catchphrase.

But it wasn't until I launched *Eat This, Not That!* in 2007 that real change began to happen. The first of nearly twenty books in the Eat This, Not That! franchise said it all in the dedication, when my coauthor Matt Goulding and I called out Applebee's, Olive Garden, Outback, Red Lobster, and T.G.I. Friday's for concealing their nutritional information. (Today, each and every one provides full nutritional data for all their offerings.)

At first, food manufacturers hated me. But soon, they began to change their tune. When we ran a blog in 2008 exposing Baskin-Robbins for producing a 2,310-calorie Heath Bar milkshake, the company followed up by scrapping the drink, as well as its entire line of "premium" shakes. Jamba Juice unveiled a line of high-fructose corn syrup–free drinks in 2009, and CEO James White cited Eat This, Not That! as the inspiration for the move. A few months later, Gatorade and Hunt's took steps to reduce HFCS and, by the end of that year, HFCS consumption in the United States began to drop for the first time in thirty years.

Few movements have changed the way we eat more than Eat This,

---

ZERO SUGAR SUCCESS STORY

Sandy Villegas, sixty-two, Monroe Township, NJ:

"My stomach is gone, and my husband lost six pounds!"

Starting weight: **142** | Two weeks later: **137**

Here's what I know to be true: I retired from my job in October and have increased my exercise since then, trying to lose some very stubborn fat around my waist. I tried Weight Watchers and lost five pounds but I know I was not eating healthy—even though I dropped some pounds—because I ate a lot of refined carbs every day. Pretty soon, I noticed two things: **1)** I was hitting a weight-loss plateau and **2)** my stomach was as bloated as ever!

Now, thanks to *Zero Sugar Diet*, my stomach is almost gone! I don't crave carbs all day and if I do have a treat, it is just that and purposely chosen. Just as important, before going on the diet, I was told I am borderline diabetic. I haven't had a glucose level of 86 and an A1C of under 6.0 in several years—but I do now, thanks to Zero Sugar. The huge drop in my lab numbers was primarily due to the changes in this way of eating. In fact, my doctor has taken me off blood pressure medication! One added bonus is that my husband has dropped six pounds as I cook for the two of us. Thanks so much, Dave!

Not That! From the world of nutritional mystery I first wrote about in 2002, we emerged in 2015 to a new day, when the FDA at last required calorie counts to be displayed in all chain restaurants and movie theaters—long after most restaurants, under pressure from ticked-off consumers, had already made the move voluntarily.

But knowing what you're eating is only part of the battle. How and when to eat is also important. I wrote *The 8-Hour Diet* in 2012 in response to shocking new research about longevity and how the timing of our meals could dramatically extend our lives, flatten our bellies, and reduce our risk of diabetes. And in 2013, I began tracking breakthrough research emerging out of Europe about nutrigenics—the study of how our genes interact with our food in ways that determine whether or not our fat genes get triggered.

The book that resulted from that research, *Zero Belly Diet*, became one of the biggest books of 2015, and it solved for me one of the great personal mysteries of my life—why my brother Eric was a star athlete in high school, while I was a flailing firkin of flab. It turns out that, like Eric and me, most of us carry the fat genes, but it's only when we eat too much of the wrong food, and too little of the right food, that those genes wake up and cause us to begin storing more fat than we want to. His healthy eating habits didn't trigger his obesity storage genes; my diet of Cheetos and Cheez Whiz did.

But *Zero Belly Diet* opened my eyes to new science that demanded further exploration. One of those breaking areas of research was the role that fiber had in feeding our gut biomes—the complex systems of bacteria that live in our digestive organs and do much more than just break down food. They play an essential role in managing our hormones, our energy levels, and even our immune systems. A balanced gut means physical and emotional health, as well as a properly calibrated sequence of genes that are firing the way nature intended. Feed the good bacteria, and you lose weight. Feed the bad, and you gain.

And guess what the bad bacteria love to eat? Sugar.

And if you've peeked ahead into this book, you can already guess what the good bacteria love to eat: fiber.

So I started to take a harder look at how sugar and fiber were accounted for in our food supply. And the truth is, marketers have dozens of clever ways to hide sugar, from obscuring which sugars are added and which are natural, to adding a variety of sugars and then listing them separately on the label, so no one form of sugar appears too high up on the ingredients list. (Don't be surprised to find that some products use cane syrup, cane sugar, molasses, brown sugar, corn syrup, and more, all at the same time.)

How the Food Industry Is Aligned Against Us

To find out why sugar was showing up in such enormous quantities in places like Sonic Onion Rings (51 grams in a family-size order), P.F. Chang's Sesame Chicken (76 grams of sugar), and Cheesecake Factory Teriyaki Chicken (96 grams per serving), I decided to dial up the manufacturers and see what they had to say for themselves. We reached out to forty different brands and asked them pointedly why they were adding so much sugar to their foods. (Their responses are on page 62.) I guarantee you'll come away ready to organize a march on your local Domino Sugar factory.

The research that informed this book revealed new ways in which our American food industry is undermining our quest for flatter bellies and healthier, happier lives. Worse, it revealed how many food marketers were able to find loopholes in the new regulations for nutritional transparency. Some chain restaurants, such as T.G.I. Friday's and Ruby Tuesday, don't list sugar content as part of their nutritional data. Others, like Starbucks, provide it for their beverages but not their foods.

And we're not making nearly the dent in our sugar intake as we'd like, for just these reasons. HFCS consumption started to drop in the early 2000s, a decline accelerated by the attention Eat This, Not That! was bringing to this artificially manufactured source of sugar calories.

(You'll read why HFCS is particularly harmful in a later chapter.) But as our HFCS intake has dropped, our consumption of refined cane and beet sugar has started to rise again, according to the USDA—in part because, even as we start to eschew sodas and other HFCS-sweetened drinks, food makers are adding more natural sugars to our salads, our sandwiches, and our soups. As a nation, we took in 352 sugar calories per person per day in 2013, about 75 percent more than the USDA recommends.

THE BITTER TRUTH ABOUT SWEETS

In early 2016, I conducted a poll of 271 people to see how they felt about sugar. I figured I'd get some funny responses, along the lines of "Where's the chocolate factory, Mr. Wonka?"

What I didn't expect was to discover a population that feels angry and powerless before the allure of sugar, one that's wracked with guilt to such a degree that the majority go out of their way to hide their sugar obsessions. Here's what I found; see if you don't recognize yourself in these statistics.

We crave sweets (of course)

When we asked folks, "When you get a food craving, what are you most likely to crave?"

54.4 percent said sugary foods.

35.2 percent said salty foods.

10.4 percent said fatty foods.

Cake, chocolate, cookies, and ice cream—and often some combination of those four—were the top crave-worthy foods, with doughnuts, baked goods, and candy making solid showings.

We can't resist them

47 percent of respondents say they can't have sweets around the house without eating them.

And we feel bad about it . . .

68.4 percent of respondents say they've felt guilty after eating a sugary food.

. . . So we hide it

29 percent of respondents confessed that they have hidden sugary sweets around the house so they could eat them unobserved.

My Own Struggle with Sugar

If you asked twenty-five-year-old me to predict what my forties would look like, I would have used just one word to describe them: fat.

Fat was my inevitable destiny; how could it not be? I had grown up as a lonely, latchkey kid with a serious sugar addiction; my best friends were the Three Musketeers and all I knew of the world outside my suburban Pennsylvania neighborhood was French vanilla, English tof-

---

. . . Or we freak out.

When dealing with guilt around sweets, some respondents say they'll stop eating for the day; toss their sugary foods in the trash; binge on exercise; or simply make pledges never to indulge again:

"I promise myself I will cut back on sugar and try to avoid sugary foods (but it doesn't usually work)."

"Restrict calories the next days."

"Cry, then try to compensate with the next meal."

"Get mad at myself, then drink water."

"Try to talk myself into better self-control."

"Hide the wrapper."

"Go to the gym and work off the 500 calories."

"Sulk."

"Isolate."

"Just feel bad, and sometimes eat more because I feel bad."

Meals don't feel complete without sugary foods

44.4 percent say that when they finish dinner, they don't feel satisfied unless they've had dessert.

22.3 percent regularly eat something sweet for breakfast or with their coffee.

We use sugar to quench our thirst

52 percent of respondents drink at least one sweetened beverage a day.

27.5 percent drink two to four sweetened beverages a day.

And our blood sugar is out of control

92.1 percent crave chocolate or something sweet at least once a day.

42.3 percent say they get cravings more than once a day.

63.3 percent say they've experienced a "sugar rush" followed by a crash.

65.2 percent report often feeling fatigued and craving something sweet in the afternoon.

fee, and Dutch chocolate. When my lumpy, loafy two hundred pounds went lumbering into the Navy Reserves after college, I could see the disgust on the face of the basic training instructors: Who sent us this leaky old tugboat? And how the heck are we supposed to turn it into a battleship?

The Navy did whip me into shape—morning revelry of burpees and wind sprints for months on end will do that to you—but when I entered the workforce soon after, the weight began to pile back on. To fight back, I started exercising like a fiend, completing the New York Marathon twice and turning the company gym into an extension of my office.

But in a lot of ways, I was just trying to outrun the devil. My father had struggled with severe obesity for most of his own adulthood—he'd be dead from a weight-related stroke by the time he was fifty-two— and there was no reason to believe that destiny wasn't awaiting me, too. I tried to eat healthily, but no matter how hard I exercised, nothing could overcome my own desires for sweet, instantly gratifying confections.

As I gained success in my career, first as the editor in chief of *Men's Health* and founder of Eat This, Not That!, and later as the editorial director of *Men's Fitness* and *Shape*, I learned a great deal about how to eat properly. I learned about good fats and bad fats, about the role of protein in helping us burn unwanted flab, about how to time my meals to ensure I was getting the maximum muscle-building bene- fits of each and every morsel. And as that body of knowledge grew, so, too, did my ability to help others lose weight and live healthier, happier lives.

But I was still exercising like a fiend, because I was still a slave to my sweet tooth. I'd struggle to stay awake during long afternoon meetings, longing to get back to my office for a cup of coffee and a chocolate-coated energy bar. I figured my destiny was to sweat through my gym clothes day after day; it was the only way I'd stay healthy and in shape.

And then I came across a bit of research that changed everything. And I learned that while I had, indeed, been doing almost everything right, the fact was, I was trying too hard. Weight loss was easier than any of us ever imagined.

In 2015, researchers at the University of Massachusetts compared two sets of dieters. One set had spent the previous year doing pretty much everything that I did: cut calories, reduced saturated fat, ate lots of fruits and vegetables, took the skin off their chicken, ate low-fat dairy items, cut sodium, ate more fish, reduced trans fats, cut back on sugar, and exercised a minimum of 150 minutes a week. The other group did none of those things. All they did was to eat more fiber, at least 30 grams a day.

Yet after a year, both groups showed nearly identical reductions in weight, blood pressure, cholesterol levels, blood sugar, and inflammation.

My first reaction? I was mad. Car-flipping mad.

I had spent years working hard, depriving myself, battling my cravings, and for what? I could have simply been eating more fiber, thereby balancing my hunger hormones, calming my sweet tooth, and losing weight without all the sweat.

I dove deeper into the research, and as I did, I began adding more fiber into my own day. I discovered how incredibly easy it was to stop hunger in its tracks and, even better, to put an end to the energy lulls and cravings that had haunted me since my youth. My stomach became defined in a way that I hadn't seen since my New York Marathon days, and I was laser-focused both at work and at home.

But more important, I had begun to unravel the mystery of why we're so much heavier today than we were back in the 1980s, and how we could all begin enjoying easy, automatic weight loss without so much desperate effort.

As I began to teach others this simple method of nutritional balance, I saw how quickly they could see dramatic results. Within just two weeks of rethinking their fiber/sugar intake, their bodies, and their daily lives, had changed for the better.

Now, I'm going to teach this revolutionary new program to you.

AN OPEN LETTER FROM
YOUR PANCREAS

Dear Friend:

Ours has been a long and fruitful collaboration. And hence it pains me to write this missive, but I fear I have no choice.

You and I have been a team since day one. Indeed, our very first gulp of milk from Mom began a relationship that has benefited us both in innumerable ways. You were always the face of our brand—and yes, the arms, legs, and hair as well. Me, I was happy to toil away down in the bowels of the operation, doing the dirty work, pumping digestive juices into your duodenum.

Quite frankly, it's been a thankless job. Those ribs and cornbread muffins you're so enamored of? By the time they reach me they're just a goopy, glutinous mass of partially digested carbs, raw protein and fat, and stomach acids. And some leftover spit. It's pretty gross, really. I mean, when do I get to taste the barbecue sauce, or wash down a meal with a cold beer? Um, never, that's when. But you need me to digest proteins, carbs, and fat. Without me, nothing happens down here. And so I toil on.

But that's not all I do. My Islets of Langerhans—which, by the way, I get zero maintenance help from you on—pump out insulin to manage your blood sugar. Insulin, as you well know, is the hormone that turns the glucose in your blood into either energy or, increasingly—and please don't take this as a personal attack—belly fat. Yes, you're the one with the insulin receptors, but I'm the one sending the messages. You don't get all the credit just for signing the delivery slip, you know!

And here's where I need to stand up and say,
Enough.

Just the other night, I joined you on the couch
for an episode of *Modern Family*, except that
it was a repeat, so you started surfing around
like you do when you're bored, and we wound up
watching the last half of *Undercover Boss*. And
because you were bored, you ripped open that
box of Teddy Grahams that you bought for the
kids, and the next thing you know, it's O'Hare
Airport at Christmastime down here. Sugar all
over the place, and I'm pumping out insulin
like mad. And when my insulin finally corrals
the sugar and gets it to your receptor cells,
it's like, "Sorry, dude, we're closing up."
I had to send extra insulin just to break down
the doors of your lazy-ass receptors to deliver
the package.

And that's when it struck me: These poor,
anonymous, underpaid, overworked employees on
Undercover Boss are just like me. They toil
away in obscurity, just waiting for someone to
notice how hard they're working. Well, same
here, inside your belly: Your stomach gets all
the attention, and even your colon has been
getting some video play of late. (Congrats on
the clean 'scope, by the way.) Me, I just keep
working. And all I ever hear is, "More insulin,
stat!"

Well, there is no more. You can't keep
pressing the SUGAR button and expecting me to
answer the bell. You're burning out your
insulin receptors, and you're burning me out
as well. Starting tonight, I'll be reducing
my insulin output. I just don't have it in me
anymore. And your blood sugar? Well, that's
your problem.

chapter 2

THE
#1 HEALTH
THREAT
IN AMERICA

HERE'S A QUICK QUESTION: How many spoonfuls of high-fructose corn syrup did you eat yesterday?

Oh, you don't recall slurping down any of the hyper-sweet corn extract? Well, you did—about eight teaspoons' worth, according to the U.S. Department of Agriculture. In fact, the average American consumed twenty-seven pounds of the stuff last year.

But while eight teaspoons of artificially manufactured syrup may seem like an awful lot, it's only a drop in the sugar bucket. The USDA's most recent figures find that Americans consume, on average, about thirty-two teaspoons of added sugar every single day. That sugar comes to us in the form of candies, ice cream, and other desserts, yes.

But the most troubling sugar of all isn't the added sugar we consume on purpose; it's the stuff we don't even know we're eating.

In recent years, the medical community has begun to coalesce around a powerful new way of looking at added sugar: as perhaps the number one most significant health threat in America. But what exactly is "added sugar," and why do experts suddenly believe that it's the Darth Vader of nutrition?

When they talk about "added sugar," health experts aren't talking about the stuff that we consume from eating whole foods. They're talking about "free sugars," the stuff that doesn't have a fiber (or protein) accompaniment, and that makes its way into our food in the manufacturing process. So lactose, the sugar naturally found in milk and dairy products, and naturally occurring fructose, the sugar that appears in fruit, don't count. But ingredients that are used in foods to provide added sweetness and calories, from the much-maligned high-fructose corn syrup to healthier-sounding ones like agave, date syrup, cane sugar, and honey, are all considered added sugars.

But aren't all sugars created equal? Not really, say experts. Sugar comes in pretty much three forms:

Sucrose: That's table sugar to you and me. It's the granular stuff in Grandma's apple pie, the lump or two you add into your coffee, the fine white powder that's dusted over a deep-fried funnel cake. Sucrose is a slightly complicated molecule, so our bodies don't really want to have to deal with it. In fact, within seconds of sucrose hitting our intestines, our enzymes split it into two separate molecules: glucose and fructose.

Glucose: A simple sugar found in all carbs, glucose is used immediately by our bodies for energy, or stored in the muscles and the liver as glycogen. Glucose is the stuff that shoots directly into the bloodstream and causes our pancreas to pump out insulin; insulin pulls it out of the bloodstream so the body can use it and, if there's too much of it, stores the excess as fat.

Fructose: The body can't really use fructose for energy, at least not right away. Fructose is instead shuttled to the liver, where it's metabolized and stored as fat. This process causes spikes in the hormone ghrelin, the "I'm still hungry" hormone that sends us out seeking additional calories. Fructose behaves in the body much the way alcohol does, and has the same damaging effect on the liver; the only difference is that you don't catch a buzz.

Fructose may be the most problematic type of sugar, health-wise: according to one study, fructose may increase blood pressure, increase heart rate, and boost myocardial oxygen demand (basically, how much oxygen your heart needs to function). It may also contribute to inflammation, insulin resistance, and overall metabolic dysfunction. And we get more fructose in our diets today than was ever possible before, thanks to high-fructose corn syrup, the sweetener used in soda and most other convenience foods.

But wait: Fructose is the kind of sugar found in fruit. So isn't it healthy and natural?

Not really. It's almost impossible to eat too much fructose through natural means. Consider this: You'd need to eat six cups of strawberries to get the same amount of fructose as in one can of Coke. That's in part because high-fructose corn syrup is a type of sugar that simply doesn't exist in nature. Corn syrup itself is 100 percent glucose, but to make it sweeter, manufacturers add pure fructose until the mix is 55:45 fructose to glucose. That makes for a sweetener that's unnaturally high in the very form of sugar that has health experts so concerned.

And even if you did decide to eat six cups of strawberries, you're still not going to cause the same sort of fructose overload as you will with just one soda. That's because the fiber in strawberries (and any other fruit) helps to slow down digestion and prevent rapid blood sugar spikes. The Coke, by delivering the same amount of fructose in concentrated liquid form, creates an instant sugar high.

Your Body, on Sugar

If all the added sugars we consumed came from our nightly ice-cream cone, or the chocolate bar we stole from the kids, or maybe that tablespoon of maple syrup we threw on our pancakes this morning, that would be fine. That's how people lived a hundred years ago, and everybody's pants fit back then.

The reason it's almost impossible to stick to the USDA guidelines is because added sugars are everywhere. A woman can blow through her allotment of sugar in just one sitting, and not by ordering cake, ice cream, or cookies but by ordering a "health" food. For example, at Applebee's, a Grilled Shrimp 'N Spinach Salad delivers 50 grams of sugar; so does an order of Sweet Potato Fries & Dips. Chili's Caribbean Salad with Grilled Chicken serves up 69 grams of sugar, while the Moroccan-Spiced Chicken Salad at California Pizza Kitchen comes with 80 grams. And at Jamba Juice, one of those Acai Primo Bowls packs 96 grams of sugar. Taking it to a whole new level is Smoothie King, which offers on their "Fitness Blends" menu a line of drinks called The Hulk, made for people who want to build lean muscle. But their large strawberry version contains a stunning 1,928 calories and 250 grams of sugar—as much as an adult male should eat in five whole days.

Spinach salads? Acai bowls? Fitness smoothies? They make a couple of Snickers bars look like a healthy lunch in comparison. Even "light" foods and beverages can cause you to throw back a day's worth of sugar in a few gulps. At Starbucks, you probably think you're doing okay if you order the "Light" version of their Java Chip Frappuccino, but even this drink weighs in at 46 grams of sugar for a Venti version. (At least that's better than the 88 grams in their regular Java Chip!)

It ticks you off. It ticks me off. And I realized I had to do something.

That's why giving fourteen days can make such a difference

One study already proved it: People who consume beverages containing high-fructose corn syrup for two weeks significantly increased their levels of triglycerides and LDL cholesterol (the "bad" cholesterols), plus two proteins associated with elevated cholesterols and another compound, uric acid, that's associated with diabetes and gout, reported *The American Journal of Clinical Nutrition* in 2015.

Terrible news? Actually, no. It's great news, and why the *Zero Sugar Diet* is such a powerful weapon in protecting you and your health. Because it proves that altering your sugar intake for just fourteen days can make a dramatic impact not only on how you look but on your current and future health.

In fact, in a 2014 editorial in the journal *JAMA Internal Medicine*, the authors made a bold statement: "Too much sugar does not just make us fat; it can also make us sick."

Just take a look at all it's doing to you.

ZERO SUGAR SUCCESS STORY

Ricky Casados, fifty-six, Albuquerque, NM:

My muscles are showing and I don't even need sweets!

Starting weight: **157** | Four weeks later: **148**

My original goal weight was 152 pounds, but now I'm down to 148! I feel really good, and have not eaten a piece of chocolate cake or cookies—my vices—since I started the diet, and my blood sugar is stable. The first week was the hardest to resist sweets but by the second week it was not a problem. Today I don't even need sweets with sugar—now it's fruits. And as a result, muscle is beginning to show again!

And just a short footnote: My wife, as of last week, has begun *Zero Sugar Diet*, after seeing me drop a few pounds, and she now also has quit sweets. Just yesterday at work, at a party for a co-worker, they brought out three different cakes along with cupcakes, and she did not touch one piece. Very proud of her.

Added sugar makes eating healthy almost impossible.

The more added sugar that sneaks its way into your diet, the less healthy food you'll eat the rest of the day. That's the finding of a 2015 article in *Nutrition Reviews*, which looked at dozens of studies conducted between 1972 and 2012. The researchers found that a higher intake of added sugar was associated with poorer diet and a lower intake of micronutrients.

That's in part because of how sugary foods retrain our taste buds and mess with our bodily systems. When even tomato sauce is laced with sweetener, we then need greater and greater doses of sugar in order for the flavor to register. That leads us to seek out candies and baked goods at the expense of real food.

But it's not just a matter of taste. A sugar rush creates an overflow of insulin into the system to try to manage the toxic substance. Because it can create an overreaction within the body—too much insulin pulling too much sugar out of the bloodstream—it can lead to a crash that sends us seeking another immediate sugar rush, the kind that no whole food can satisfy.

The most powerful effects, however, aren't on our bodies. They're on our brains. In one study, researchers measured the levels of oxytocin, a feel-good hormone that helps us feel satiated, in the brains of rats. When rats that ate a low-sugar diet were given a meal high in sugar, their oxytocin levels didn't change. But when they were given the high-sugar diet regularly, their brains began to show lower levels of oxytocin activity. In other words, the more we're bombarded with added sugars, the more chronically unsatisfied we feel, and the more we need to eat. And a similar study at New York University found that a rise in insulin—the hormone that processes blood sugar—causes a simultaneous rise in dopamine, a neurotransmitter that triggers the brain's pleasure center.

That might be why artificial sweeteners cause us to seek out additional calories, according to a 2013 study in *The Journal of Physi-*

CAN YOUR BODY SURVIVE WITHOUT SUGAR?

The old saying is "Life is sweet." But after hearing about the horrors of sugar, many people ask me, Can I live a life without sweets—altogether? For how long? And what would happen to my body?

Well, our bodies can certainly go without sugar. And our bodies can definitely go without sugar and refined grains. Life without processed sugar or refined grains would be very healthy! But can we live without carbohydrates altogether? That's a different story.

Carbohydrates are the traditional source of fuel—aka glucose— for our brains, heart, muscles, and central nervous system. Complex carbohydrates—such as whole grains—are the best source of carbohydrates and are an important part of a healthy diet. They benefit our bodies by providing fiber, vitamins, and minerals, as well as slowing the absorption of glucose and improving satiety and cholesterol levels. Without carbohydrates, the body will use protein and fat as fuel—this is called ketosis. When your body is in the metabolic state of ketosis, it turns fat into ketones in the liver, which will supply energy instead of glucose, as if you were fasting.

You may have heard of the ketogenic diet, in fact, which focuses on protein and fat intake, while maintaining a very low carbo-hydrate intake. This diet, newly trendy, may have benefits such as weight loss and improved blood sugar levels. However, it is very restrictive; eliminating healthy fruits, vegetables, legumes, and other nutritious complex carbohydrates seems unnecessary and no fun. Also, we don't know the long-term effects of ketosis (though if you do go too long without any carbs, it can lead to heart or kidney disease). What I do know, after years of studying nutrition, is that any diet that is very restrictive or eliminates entire food groups can be unrealistic and difficult to sustain. That's why *Zero Sugar Diet* eliminates added sugars—but allows natural ones. Pretty sweet deal.

ology. The study identified a specific physiological brain signal that actually helps us determine the difference between real and artificial sweeteners; the signal trips our dopamine factory, but only when it determines that we're actually getting sugar calories.

An editorial in *JAMA Internal Medicine* asked, "Why Are We Consuming So Much Sugar Despite Knowing Too Much Can Harm Us?" The answer: "The high prevalence of added-sugar consumption . . . is very likely influenced by and a result of addictive behaviors incited by reward system activation after overeating highly palatable foods."

Added sugar causes your body to store fat around your belly.

Within twenty-four hours of eating fructose, your body is flooded with elevated levels of triglycerides. Does that sound bad? It is.

Triglycerides are the fatty deposits in your blood. Your liver makes them, because they're essential for building and repairing the tissues in your body. But when it's hit with high doses of fructose, the liver responds by pumping out more triglycerides; that's a signal to your body that it's time to store some abdominal fat. In one study, researchers fed subjects beverages sweetened with either glucose or fructose. Both gained the same amount of weight over the next eight weeks, but the fructose group gained its weight primarily as belly fat, thanks to the way this type of sugar is processed in the liver.

What's unique to fructose is that it seems to be a universal obesogen—in other words, every creature that eats it gains weight. Princeton researchers recently found that high-fructose corn syrup seemed to have a unique impact on weight in their animal studies. The most startling finding, according to the researchers, was that 100 percent of the rats that consumed the HFCS became obese, a result not seen in other diet experiments—for example, when animals are fed high-fat diets. Fructose is the freak show of fat.

Added sugar makes you skip going to the gym.

There are a lot of ways that added sugar can make you gain weight, but the most bizarre may be the way it reduces actual physical activity. In one study at the University of Illinois, two groups of mice were followed for two and a half months; both groups were fed the same amount of sugar and calories, but one group was fed a diet that mimicked the standard American adolescent's diet—i.e., one that was about 18 percent added fructose. The other set received its sugar in the form of glucose. The added fructose group gained more body fat over the course of the study, even though they weren't fed more calories—or even more sugar. One of the reasons was that the fructose-addled mice traveled about 20 percent less in their little cages than the other set of mice. They just naturally . . . slowed . . . down.

Added sugar is a primary driver in your risk of dying from diabetes.

The link between increased sugar and diabetes risk is right up there with "smoking causes lung cancer" on the list of immutable medical truths—despite what soda manufacturers are trying to tell us. (You'll read more about sugar-based hocus-pocus in the next chapter.) But researchers at the Mayo Clinic have come right out and said that added fructose—either as a constituent of table sugar or as the main component of high-fructose corn syrup—may be the number one cause of diabetes, and that cutting sugar alone could translate into a reduced number of diabetes deaths the world over.

Added sugar makes you dumb, demented, and depressed.

"Reduce fructose in your diet if you want to protect your brain," announced Fernando Gomez-Pinilla, professor at the University of California, Los Angeles. He and his team tested how well rats recovering from brain injury learned new ways to get through a maze. They found that animals that drank HFCS took 30 percent more time to find the exit. "Our findings suggest that fructose disrupts plasticity—the creation of fresh pathways between brain cells that occurs when we learn or experience something new," he says.

In an earlier study, researchers found that a combination of sugar and fat could actually change one's brain chemistry. The brains of animals on a high-fat, high-sugar diet had decreased levels of brain-delivered neurotropic factor (BDNF), a compound that helps brain cells communicate with one another, build memories, and learn new things; decreased levels of BDNF have been linked to both Alzheimer's and depression.

One of the recent mysteries of science is why depression, diabetes, and dementia seem to cluster in epidemiological studies, and why having one of these health issues seems to increase your risk for the others. The answer: In a study in the journal *Diabetologia*, researchers found that when blood glucose levels are elevated, BDNF levels drop. That means that the simple act of eating sugar makes you instantly dumber; the more you do it, the greater your risk of diabetes, and the greater your risk of depression and dementia as well. In a 2015 study of post-menopausal women, higher levels of added sugars and refined carbs were associated with an increased likelihood of depression, while higher consumption of fiber, dairy, fruit, and vegetables was associated with a lower risk.

And, in a study of nearly one thousand seniors (median age: 79.5), researchers found that eating a diet high in simple carbs significantly increased the risk of developing dementia. All of the subjects were cognitively normal at the beginning of the study, and about two hundred developed signs of dementia over the next 3.7 years. The risk of mental decline was higher in those who ate high-carb diets, and lower in those whose diets were higher in fat and/or protein.

WHY "SUGAR-FREE" ISN'T THE ANSWER

If the key to weight loss were simply to cut down on sugar, this would be a very short book, indeed. All you'd need to do is to drink diet soda, eat sugar-free cookies, and opt for "lite" syrup on your pancakes. Toss a few packets of Splenda in your coffee and you're good.

But it doesn't work that way—not by a long shot.

We are, after all, a fickle and complicated species, and our bodies react to foods in ways we can't always predict. For example, when we eat or drink something that tastes sweet, our brains get all psyched to digest sugar. The brain signals the pancreas to create more insulin, so as to better manage the sugar calories it's anticipating.

So what happens when those calories don't come? Scientists are still trying to understand the exact fallout, but some studies have indicated that over time, this process can impair the body's ability to react properly to insulin, which primes you for diabetes.

What we do know about artificial sweeteners, however, isn't particularly good:

Artificial sweeteners cause belly fat . . .
A 2015 study in the *Journal of the American Geriatrics Society* found that increasing diet soda intake is directly linked to greater abdominal obesity. In a study of older adults, researchers found that those who drank diet soda daily experienced more than triple the increase in waist size over the course of nine years.

. . . And change how your brain works.
In 2012, researchers reporting in the journal *Physiology & Behavior* discovered that the brains of those who drink diet sodas regularly react differently to sweet tastes than those who don't have regular doses of artificial sweeteners. The scientists gave young adults drinks containing either sugar or saccharin. Afterward, their brains were examined using MRIs.

Sugar doubles your risk of
dying from heart disease.

People who get 25 percent or more of their calories from added sugar are more than twice as likely to die from heart disease as those who eat less than 10 percent, according to a study in *JAMA: The Journal of the American Medical Association*. One out of ten of us falls into that category.

Now, if you're an average American, your daily sugar consumption is about 17 percent of calories, according to the study. But that's hardly a laurel to rest on. People who ate between 17 and 21 percent of their calories from added sugar had a 38 percent higher risk of dying from heart disease, compared with people who consumed 8 percent or less of their calories from added sugar.

At first, the researchers figured that since those who ingest more sugar have poorer diets, that might be a main cause. But even after making adjustments for the quality of one's diet, the link between sweets and cardiovascular risk remained the same.

The study found that the major sources of added sugar in the American diet were:

- ▶ Sugar-sweetened beverages **(37.1 percent)**
- ▶ Grain-based desserts like cookies or cake **(13.7 percent)**
- ▶ Fruit drinks **(8.9 percent)**
- ▶ Dairy desserts like ice cream **(6.1 percent)**
- ▶ Candy **(5.8 percent)**

And sodas and other sweet drinks are a major red flag: The researchers found that a higher consumption of sugar-sweetened beverages was directly tied to an increased risk of dying from heart disease.

In a 2015 study in Sweden, researchers followed 42,400 men over the course of twelve years. They found that men who consumed at least two servings per day of sweetened beverages had a 23 percent higher risk of heart failure compared with those who did not. The impact is so great that you don't need to be meandering through middle

Researchers found that those who had consumed the saccharin drinks demonstrated greater activation of the brain sensors that react to sweet tastes. But more important, they found that those who regularly consumed diet sodas seemed to have impaired dopamine response—the "feel good" hormone that's released when we do something pleasurable, like eat delicious food.

. . . And rot your teeth.

Scientists at Melbourne University's Oral Health Cooperative Research Centre tested a wide range of sugar-free soft drinks, sports drinks, and sweets and found that many of them can cause just as much damage to one's teeth as their sugary cousins. The researchers tested fifteen soft drinks on healthy human teeth and found that all of them led to significant erosion of dental enamel. Sugar-free foods can strip away a tooth's outer layer, creating a tooth that's easily pitted and discolored. The main culprit: phosphoric acid from colas and citric acid found in lemon- or lime-flavored drinks.

. . . And harm your heart.

In a 2012 study in *The American Journal of Clinical Nutrition*, researchers found that those who drank diet beverages had higher fasting glucose, thicker waists, lower HDL (good) cholesterol, higher triglycerides, and higher blood pressure.

. . . And mess with your gut health.

A 2014 study published in the journal *Nature* found that saccharin alters the microbial balance in the gut, creating a scenario that can potentially lead to obesity and diabetes. The study was conducted on both mice and men, and found that after eleven weeks of drinking water flavored with a number of different artificial sweeteners, those mice that consumed saccharine in particular showed abnormally high glucose levels in their blood after eating.

In a separate study, researchers compared 40 people who reported eating artificial sweeteners to 236 people who did not; those who said they ate artificial sweeteners were more likely to have metabolism issues, including higher blood glucose levels.

One thing that concerns some scientists is that the artificial sweeteners we're now consuming are radically more sweet

age to see the impact: Even teenagers who consume food and beverages high in added sugars show evidence of risk factors for heart disease and diabetes in their blood, according to a second study in *The Journal of Nutrition*.

Added sugar raises your blood pressure.

In fact, sugar may be worse for your blood pressure than salt, according to a paper published in the journal *Open Heart*. Just a few weeks on a high-sucrose diet can increase both systolic and diastolic blood pressure. Another study found that for every sugar-sweetened beverage, risk of developing hypertension increased 8 percent. Too much sugar leads to higher insulin levels, which in turn activate the sympathetic nervous system and lead to increased blood pressure, according to James J. DiNicolantonio, PharmD, cardiovascular research scientist at Saint Luke's Mid America Heart Institute in Kansas City, Missouri. "It may also cause sodium to accumulate within the cell, causing calcium to build up within the cell, leading to vasoconstriction and hypertension," he says.

Sugar causes your skin to sag.

Your skin has its own support system in the form of collagen and elastin, two compounds that keep your skin tight and plump. But when elevated levels of glucose and fructose enter the body, they link to the amino acids present in the collagen and elastin, producing advanced glycation end products, or "AGEs." That damages these two critical compounds and makes it hard for the body to repair them. This process is accelerated in the skin when sugar is elevated, and further stimulated by ultraviolet light, according to a study in *Clinical Dermatology*. In other words, eating lots of sugar poolside is the worst thing you can do for your skin.

This wreaks havoc on our system. When our body gets out of bal-

than traditional flavorings like aspartame and saccharin. Here's a look at the chemicals currently approved for use by the Food and Drug Administration:

Aspartame (Equal, NutraSweet): 180X sweeter than sugar
Found in: diet sodas, teas, coffee flavorings, energy drinks, protein shakes, flavored milk, juices, high-fiber cereals, flavored water

Acesulfame-K (Sunett, Sweet One): 200X sweeter
Found in: Soft drinks, fruit juices, alcoholic beverages, dairy, ice cream, jellies and preserves, baked goods, gum, marinated fish, breakfast cereals, processed fruits and vegetables, salad dressings, condiments and relishes, soups

SGFE (Nectresse): 100–250X sweeter
An extract from the Chinese monk fruit or Luo Han Guo fruit found in: frozen desserts, soft drinks

Saccharin (Sweet'N Low, Necta Sweet): 300X sweeter
"Lite" salad dressings, candies, dessert toppings, jams and jellies, canned fruit

Stevia (Truvia, PureVia): 200–400X sweeter
Found in: teas, candies, chewing gum, soft drinks, soy sauce

Sucralose (Splenda): 600X sweeter
Soft drinks, iced teas and coffees, juice drinks, flavored syrups, chewing gum, protein drinks, energy bars, baked goods, ice cream, gummy bears, microwave popcorn

Neotame: 7,000–13,000X sweeter
Approved in 2002, it's found in: carbonated soft drinks, powdered soft drinks, baked goods, dairy, chewing gum

Advantame: 20,000X sweeter
Newly approved in 2014, it's found in: dairy drinks, frozen desserts, beverages, chewing gum

ance, it wants to reach out for something to stabilize it. That something is usually packed with fat and carbohydrates—comfort foods like mac & cheese, or quick energy sources like cake or cookies. (By the way, that's not going to change; if that's what your body wants, that's what your body is going to get, and no amount of discipline is going to change that. I'll show you why that's okay, and teach you how to eat those foods safely so you can remain healthy, lean, and in balance.)

Our weight balance—whether we're comfortably lean or grasping frantically for quick energy—is determined primarily by two hormones, called ghrelin and leptin. Leptin is the "satiety" hormone. Your body secretes leptin to tell your brain that your energy tank is topped off, you've had enough to eat, and there's no reason to go back to the buffet for thirds. When you're healthy, this hormone is balanced against ghrelin, the "feed me" hormone.

But in our modern-day walk toward weight loss, our hormones are in rebellion. Leptin is created by your fat cells; when they begin to shrink, they produce less of the "I'm good" hormone. Thanks to the lower levels of leptin, your brain gets overwhelmed by ghrelin, which transmits the message that there's not enough energy stored in your body, and your tank is on "E." And so it sends you on the search for more calories. In fact, you're more likely to overeat when you start to lose weight because your brain has become less sensitive to the signals from the gut saying that you've eaten enough.

In other words, as soon as we find the right energy balance and start losing weight, our bodies try to knock us off balance again. "The vast majority of individuals who attempt to lose weight are not able to achieve and maintain [even] a 10% reduction over a year," according to a 2015 study in the journal *Obesity Reviews*. The researchers found that even when we do succeed in losing weight, more than a third of that weight returns within a year, and almost all of it is gained back within three to five years. That's because losing weight, and keeping it off, isn't just about controlling our food intake. It's about controlling the hormones that fall out of balance, telling us to overeat and preventing us from dropping pounds.

Zero Sugar Diet will show you how to use your body's hormone cycles to eradicate hunger, by helping you eat more food—and slowing the signaling of these hormones so you never feel hungry or in need of more energy than your body can use. You'll do it by using a simple strategy that protects your body from the effects of sugar—a strategy that will allow you to eat your favorite foods, without gaining weight and without putting yourself at risk for disease.

chapter 3

TOWARD
A NEW WAY
OF EATING

WE ALL WANT TO EAT A "BALANCED DIET." But what does the term "balanced diet" even mean nowadays, when we're given so many nutritional instructions from so many sources all at the same time? We're supposed to cut down on saturated fat, eat more fish, get eight servings of vegetables a day, drink eight glasses of water, have a gram of protein for every pound of body weight, avoid gluten, cut down on carbs, reduce sodium, put butter in our coffee, make sure everything is organic and grass-fed, and still find a way to squeeze in the new superfood of the day—from coconut nectar to acai extract to avocado oil. That would be *Mission: Impossible* if we spent all of our days just thinking about our own food intake. But we've got to do it while working a full-time job and managing a social life and dealing with everything from lactose intolerance to office parties to a backseat full of cranky kids who want their Happy Meal *rightnoworelse*!

Zero Sugar Diet will teach you how to overcome all of these factors—the outside factors of our food and our society and the hormonal factors inside your own body and brain. It does so by confronting the two main issues that are making weight loss so difficult, and that set our own bodies against us:

▶ Our food has too much sugar.
▶ Our food has too little fiber.

Indeed, our sugar/fiber balance is completely out of whack, and as a result, so are our bodies.

And it's getting harder and harder each day to bring our diets back into balance. A 2015 study in *The Lancet Diabetes & Endocrinology* journal found that 74 percent of packaged foods and beverages in the United States contain caloric sweeteners, from hundreds of different versions of sugar, all of which have the same debilitating health impact. Barry Popkin, PhD, professor of nutrition at the University of North Carolina, has been cataloging packaged foods since 2007, and he and his team have assembled a mind-blowing list of 1.2 million packaged foods sold in U.S. stores that contain added sugar.

Fortunately, the U.S. Food and Drug Administration has finally stepped up and given us useful tools in our battle against added sugars. By early summer of 2018, most packaged foods sold in the United States will carry the new FDA food label, which requires listing not just the fat, calories, protein, and sugar in the food, but a more important and detailed point as well—the amount of added sugar in the food. (Other upgrades include larger, easier-to-spot calorie totals and newly added vitamin D and potassium counts, two nutrients that most Americans are deficient in.)

THESE FRUITS AND FRUIT CONCENTRATES WILL NOW COUNT AS "ADDED SUGAR"

apple
acerola
apple cider
apricot
aronia
aronia berry
banana
blackberry
black cherry
black currant
blood orange
blueberry
boysenberry
cantaloupe
carambola
cherry
chokeberry
clementine
coconut
cranberry
currant

date
dewberry
elderberry
fig
goji berry
gooseberry
grape
grapefruit
guanabana
guava
honeydew
huckleberry
kiwi
lingonberry
loganberry
lychee
mandarin orange
mango
mangosteen
marionberry
melon

mulberry
nectarine
orange
papaya
passion fruit
peach
pear
pineapple
pink grapefruit
plum
pomegranate
prune
raisin
raspberry
soursop
strawberry
tangerine
watermelon
youngberry

This is an enormous step forward for anyone worried about his or her health and weight, and it will make following the guidelines of *Zero Sugar Diet* even easier. Dairy foods come with their own natural sugars, called lactose, while whole, healthy fruits and some vegetables contain fructose. But where do those natural sugars end and the added sugars begin? With the new nutrition labels, you'll be able to compare two containers of yogurt or canned fruit and see immediately which ones contain added sugars. And it's not just cane sugar you need to look out for. Everything from molasses to agave nectar to evaporated apple juice is, in fact, an added sugar—and just as bad for you as a cube of the white stuff.

Indeed, "People are going to be shocked by the actual amount of sugar that's being added to their food," says Popkin. And many of these products seem, at first glance, pretty healthy. "The FDA does a really crude job with added sugar, for two reasons," says Popkin. "First, the current regulations exclude fruit juice concentrate." So your iced tea drink or cookie may include a certain amount of high-fructose corn syrup or cane sugar or honey in it that's counted as part of the total sugar content. But it may also include apple juice concentrate or crystallized pineapple juice that's just as sugary, but not figured into the total sugar count.

"Second, the current measurement systems are crude," Popkin says. The new labels will include fruit juice and fruit juice concentrate for the first time. As a result, foods that carry labels like "all-natural" or even "organic," but which are sweetened with fructose-based con-centrates, will be forced to show their true nature—and they won't look very natural at all.

Now, throughout this book, I've told you why you shouldn't worry about eating as much fruit as you'd like, even though fruit is high in sugar. That's because fruit is packed with fiber (as well as other critical nutrients), which helps to balance out the sugar quotient. But once you turn the fruit into juice, you strip away that healthy fiber; then, by concentrating it, you crank the sugar volume up even more.

THESE SOMETIMES "HEALTHY"-SOUNDING SUGARS ARE NOTHING MORE THAN ADDED SUGAR

agave juice
agave nectar
agave sap
agave syrup
beet sugar
brown rice syrup
brown sugar
cane juice
cane sugar
cane syrup
clintose
confectioners' powdered sugar
confectioners' sugar
corn glucose syrup
corn sweetener
corn syrup
date sugar
dextrose
drimol
dri mol
dri-mol
drisweet
dri sweet
dri-sweet
dried raisin sweetener
edible lactose
flo malt
flo-malt
flomalt

fructose
fructose sweetener
glaze and icing sugar
glaze icing sugar
golden syrup
gomme
granular sweetener
granulated sugar
hi-fructose corn syrup
high fructose corn syrup
honey
honibake
honi bake
honi-bake
honi flake
honi-flake
invert sugar
inverted sugar
isoglucose
isomaltulose
kona ame
kona-ame
lactose
liquid sweetener
malt
malt sweetener
malt syrup
maltose
maple
maple sugar

maple syrup
mizu ame
mizu-ame
mizuame
molasses
nulomoline
powdered sugar
rice syrup
sorghum
sorghum syrup
starch sweetener
sucanat
sucrose
sucrovert
sugar beet
sugar invert
sweet n neat
table sugar
treacle
trehalose
tru sweet
turbinado sugar
versatose

Courtesy of
Barry Popkin, PhD

That's why all of these diet rules—some of them scientific, others specious—are so difficult to follow. As the author of more than twenty books on food and nutrition, and a guy who spends every day reading the latest studies, nutritional theories, and breakthrough plans, I can probably name five dozen "rules" of good nutrition, just off the top of my head. But I can't follow them all—and neither can you.

Zero Sugar Diet is built on a single, simple premise: For the first fourteen days, avoid all added sugars. Then, after that, make sure your foods have less sugar than fiber. That's the "Sweet Spot," a dietary safety zone that will protect you from all of the damage that sugar can do. When you're in the sweet spot, you're getting the carbohydrates you need to run your body and your brain, and the fiber you need to keep those carbohydrates moving through your body slowly, ensuring that there's no sugar rush that sends your body into a frenzy of fat storage.

Whole foods like fruits, vegetables, and whole, unprocessed grains are in the safety zone because they have no added sugar. But when it comes to processed foods, you'll find added sugar lurking everywhere, from pasta sauce to yogurt to hot dogs. That's why I've created an extensive list of approved grocery and restaurant foods that have no added sugar, at the back of this book.

To balance out your meals, I'll have you add in Power Proteins— lean, healthy, satisfying, sugar-free foods like eggs, turkey, chicken, and fish—and Flat Belly Fats (like sugar-free salad dressings and gua- camole), which will help to heal your body and keep you satiated as your body quickly detoxes.

For two weeks, you'll observe an easy-to-follow regimen designed to retrain your taste buds, clean your system, and set your hormones back in balance. Then, you'll discover how easy it is to apply these lessons to everyday life, with a maintenance plan that looks very much like the way you enjoy eating now, but without the hunger, cravings, sugar crashes, and weight gain.

With a quick calculation you can do in your head or on your phone, you can instantly tell whether an individual food or a meal makes sense, just by measuring sugar grams against fiber grams. The brilliance of this plan is that you don't need to worry about following it perfectly. Your goal is simply to stay in the Sweet Spot, by following the program outlined in this book, and by reading the labels of packaged foods in your pantry. Just keep this rule in mind at all times after the first fourteen days:

<LOW   HIGH>
Sugar   Fiber

As long as you keep the fiber number at least as big as the sugar number, you win!

The Most Effective Diet of All Time

Your path to a lean waist and better health is only two weeks away. In fact, two weeks might be a few days longer than we need.

Earlier in this chapter, I mentioned the study that found how increasing your sugar intake for just fourteen days could have a dramatic negative impact on your health.

But what about removing sugar from your diet, even for just a short period of time? In fall of 2015, Dr. Robert Lustig, a child-obesity specialist and professor of pediatrics at the University of California, San Francisco, set out to find the answer. In a study sponsored by the National Institutes of Health and published in the journal *Obesity,* he and his team removed all added sugars from the diets of forty-three children between the ages of nine and eighteen for nine days. Each of the children selected for the study was considered at risk of diabetes and related metabolic disorders, and got an average of 27 percent of their daily calories from sugar. (By comparison, the average American adult takes in about 15 percent of calories from added sugar.)Now, as I'll tell you again and again throughout this book, reducing added sugars and adding fiber will lead to fast and dramatic weight loss. But Dr. Lustig wanted to study *only* the impact of removing sugar (remember his warning about studying one variable at a time?). His worry was that critics could say that whatever results he showed were impacted by the kids' weight loss, not by their cutting sugar. So he replaced the subjects' added sugars with starchy, low-fiber carbs, and kept their calories the same, so the kids wouldn't lose weight. Instead of yogurts sweetened with sugar, they ate bagels. Instead of pastries, they ate baked potato chips. In other words, they didn't go on a health kick: Everything about the kids' diets stayed exactly the same, including total calories, carbs, fats, and sodium. The only thing that changed was that they stopped eating added sugar.

Yet after just nine days, the kids' LDL cholesterol dropped an average of 10 points; diastolic blood pressure fell 5 points; triglycerides, the blood fat associated with heart disease, dropped 33 points. They also showed improvements in fasting blood sugar and insulin levels.

ZERO SUGAR SUCCESS STORY

Tara Anderson, forty-two, Leonardo, NJ:

"My migraines stopped and I'm no longer sick!"

Starting weight: **185** | Four weeks later: **175**

I have continued with the Zero Sugar lifestyle, and I feel really good and I find it very easy to follow. What I love about it is the way it's retrained my taste buds. I have had a little sugar a few times and it's *way* too sweet now. (I'm still trying to get used to coffee without sugar!) The best part for me is not feeling sick anymore or having migraines. It has been an all-around positive experience for me. Thank you again!

So if there's so much evidence that sugar is bad for us, why do food manufacturers keep sticking it in places where it doesn't belong? Why isn't the government doing anything to protect us?

And what the heck can we do about it?

Start *Zero Sugar Diet*, a plan that allows you to achieve perfect balance through maximum flexibility.

All I ask is that you give me fourteen days to put your body back in balance. Once you do, staying lean for the rest of your life will be easy.

ARE YOU A SUGAR ADDICT?

Why is sugar in everything nowadays? Perhaps it's because food manufacturers know that chronic exposure to sugar causes real chemical changes in the brain. Our brains need a steady supply of sugar to function. But sugar is like oxygen—too much gets you high, and then kills you.

From the moment we try sugar as a young child, our brains are rewired to crave it. Even the American Medical Association says that we overeat sugar as "a result of addictive behaviors." The more sugar we eat, the more we reduce our brain's ability to produce oxytocin, the "feel-good" hormone that tells us when we're sated. Just like with any drug, we need more of it to feel "normal" again. Answer these questions to decide whether you are, in fact, an addict.

Do you eat sweets even if you're not particularly hungry, but because you have a craving for them?

1. Rarely
2. Occasionally
3. Frequently
4. Daily

In a 2015 study at the Massachusetts Institute of Technology, researchers found that "compulsive sugar consumption is mediated by a different neural circuit than physiological, healthy eating." In other words, you may plan out balanced, healthy meals throughout the week, but that won't stop you from digging into the pantry to find a box of cookies, because the brain system that makes conscious, healthy choices is entirely different from the one that sends you scampering into the Skittles.

**Do you ever find yourself binging on sweets,
feeling cravings for sugar, or experiencing withdrawal
symptoms when you can't get your hands on them?**

> 1. **Rarely**
>
> 2. **Occasionally**
>
> 3. **Frequently**
>
> 4. **Daily**

Binging, withdrawal, and craving are the three stages of addiction, according to the American Psychiatric Association. It boils down to this: If you overeat sugar on more than a very occasional basis, or if you ever feel anxious when you can't get your hands on it, you may be struggling with addiction.

**Do you have concerns about, or have you ever been
treated for, drug or alcohol abuse?**

> **Yes**
>
> **No**

People who develop dependencies on one type of drug are more susceptible to developing dependencies on other substances—for example, alcoholics are more at risk for becoming addicted to prescription pain medication than the general public. This is known as "cross-sensitization." And because sugar affects neural pathways in a similar way to drugs, those of us who have experienced immoderation in one thing can easily become overeaters of sweets. Animal studies have shown that sugar can be a gateway to alcohol abuse. It's also been shown to be cross-addictive with both amphetamines and cocaine.

Have you ever "purged" after a sugar binge?
>   **Yes**
>   **No**

Animal studies that monitor the way the brain reacts to sugar have found that a cycle of binging and purging causes the brain to react to sugar not like a food but rather like a drug. The brain doesn't get the signal that one has stopped eating; rather, it stays geared up for more sugar.

Do you take breaks from sugar, i.e., consciously go for a day or longer without eating any sweet foods?
>   **1. Rarely**
>   **2. Occasionally**
>   **3. Frequently**
>   **4. Daily**

Cyclical binging and food deprivation may produce alterations in our brains' opioid receptors, causing us to need more of a substance to catch that buzz. That can trigger greater binging behavior.

Do you walk or drive out of your way, or get out of bed at night, in order to eat sweets?
>   **1. Rarely**
>   **2. Occasionally**
>   **3. Frequently**
>   **4. Daily**

One of the hallmarks of addiction is what researchers call "an enhanced motivation to procure an abused substance." In other words, you'll take extra steps, even destructive ones, to get your mitts on what you crave. If you notice that you're doing things to procure sweets that you wouldn't do to get other forms of food, that's a sign of addiction.

Do you feel guilty after eating sweets?
    1. Rarely
    2. Occasionally
    3. Frequently
    4. Daily

Can you think of a specific consequence of eating sweets that you've suffered (health, relationship, or job issues), but which have not deterred your sweet tooth?
    Yes
    No

Doing something that you know is unhealthy for you, and repeating the behavior over and over again, is a signal that you're not in control.

Is eating something sugary a planned activity in your day?
    1. Rarely
    2. Occasionally
    3. Frequently
    4. Daily

Do you take sugary foods with you when you go for walks or car rides?

    1. Rarely

    2. Occasionally

    3. Frequently

    4. Daily

People who are addicted to a substance will always have it on hand and will rarely venture to places where they can't get their hands on it. If you would never consider leaving the house without a treat, or going somewhere where eating wasn't a possibility, it may indicate an addiction.

Do you eat sweets alone?

    1. Rarely

    2. Occasionally

    3. Frequently

    4. Daily

Do you lie about or hide your sugary foods?

    1. Rarely

    2. Occasionally

    3. Frequently

    4. Daily

Secrecy and solitude—the compulsion to consume a substance without anyone knowing about it—is a common hallmark of any addiction. So, too, is the common behavior of creating a "stash" of something so you always have it on hand.

**Have you ever tried and failed to limit
the amount of sugar you eat?**

> **Yes**
>
> **No**

**Do you have trouble waking up in the morning
and often crash in the afternoon?**

> **1. Rarely**
>
> **2. Occasionally**
>
> **3. Frequently**
>
> **4. Daily**

Poor sleep, moodiness, poor focus, and fatigue are general symptoms of withdrawal; afternoon crashes are often a sign that you've had too much sugar earlier in the day.

SCORING YOUR SWEET TOOTH

Give yourself the corresponding numerical score for each of the multiple-choice answers above. (So if you answer Rarely, give yourself 1 point; Daily, give yourself 4 points.)

For every Yes/No answer, give yourself 4 points for Yes and 0 points for No.

10–18 points: You're not a sugar addict, just someone who has to do a bit better at watching what she eats.

19–24 points: You may well be on the verge of letting your sweet tooth run away with you. If you have a family history of addiction, you may be at special risk.

25–35 points: You're definitely eating too much sugar and, more important, you're eating it in a way that indicates you have a problem with it. If you notice cravings, fatigue, weight gain, or an inability to resist sweets even when you're trying to cut down, closely monitor both your physical and emotional state as you go through the fourteen-day cleanse, and be aware of positive changes.

36+ points: Full-blown addiction. You're probably already aware of the impact sugar is having on your life, and you've made some (unsuccessful) attempts at cutting back. *Zero Sugar Diet* will go a long way toward helping you break your addiction, but for best results, con-sider combining this program with nutritional counseling or a support group such as Overeaters Anonymous.

chapter 4

HOW TO FIND THE RIGHT SUGARS— AND AVOID THE BAD

CONSIDER THE CASE OF TWO TWENTY-FIVE-YEAR-OLD AMERICAN women. We'll call one Liz, and the other Beth.

Liz and Beth are the exact same height, follow the exact same diets, and exercise in the exact same way. They even spend their leisure time doing similar things—active stuff like biking and walking their dogs. Just about the only difference between them is that Beth loves to listen to Madonna when she dances around the house, while Liz burns calories to the sounds of Lady Gaga. But even though they eat the same amount and the same types of food, and burn off the same number of calories, Liz weighs 10 percent more than Beth does, and has a body mass index (BMI, a measure of body fat) that's 2.3 points higher.

How can that be? If our weight is determined by the calories we eat versus the calories we burn off, how can these women not weigh exactly the same?

Because there's one important difference between these two. Beth lives in America circa 1988, while Liz lives in America circa 2016. And no matter how much she diets and exercises, Liz fights a weight battle that Beth never had to face.

In fact, a person living in America today who follows the exact same diet and has the exact same degree of physical activity in her life would still weigh 10 percent more than she would have if she had been born twenty years earlier. When researchers at York University in Canada examined surveys of more than thirty-six thousand Americans, they found that today's woman exercises as much as 120 percent more than she did in the eighties, and eats about 9 percent less fat. And while we eat more carbs and total calories than we did a quarter century ago, even when the researchers adjusted for all of those factors, today's Americans were still measurably heavier.

And the damage that extra weight does is undeniable: In fact, by the time we reach forty-five, half of us have already developed pre-diabetes, an elevated blood sugar level that often precedes diabetes, according to a 2015 Harvard School of Public Health study.

The First Sugar Crash

Despite all that, sugar is not our enemy.

Our bodies run on sugar, and so do our brains. In fact, a love of sugar might be what separates us from the apes.

In a recent study in *The Quarterly Review of Biology*, researchers argue that starchy carbs played a key role in the accelerated expansion of the human brain over the past million years. They claim that the human brain uses up to 60 percent of the body's blood glucose, and that

ZERO SUGAR SUCCESS STORY

David Menkhaus, sixty-two, Liberty Township, OH:

I have type 2 diabetes and *Zero Sugar* changed my life!

Starting weight: **200** | Six weeks later: **185**

Four years ago, I was diagnosed with type 2 diabetes. For the past several years, I have been controlling my glucose levels by diet instead of medication. I took a few minutes today to analyze year-to-date daily glucose results, before and after, starting *Zero Sugar Diet*.

I test at least once a day, and sequence test time so that each condition is checked twice a week.

Reduction in Blood Glucose During Zero Sugar Diet

	Jan. 1 to Feb. 22	Feb. 23 to Apr. 16	Glucose Reduction
Fasting	119 mg/dl	111 mg/dl	8
Before Meals	102 mg/dl	98 mg/dl	4
After Meals	111 mg/dl	105 mg/dl	6
At Bedtime	121 mg/dl	101 mg/dl	20

The results above indicate that the diet has significantly lowered blood glucose levels! Not to mention, this is the easiest diet program I have ever been on:

- ▶ Easy to understand
- ▶ Easy to track
- ▶ Easy to comply
- ▶ Easy to shift between weight loss and maintenance

Thank you so much for writing this book.

once man learned to cook—unlocking the simple sugars in starches like potatoes and making them more bioavailable—it triggered evolutionary changes that increased the size of our noggins.

But it may have also triggered something else: the first sugar crash.

See, our bodies and our brains need a steady supply of sugar. And for most of our evolutionary life, we got that sugar in relatively small doses, from fiber-rich sources like fruit. With fiber as its wingman, sugar enters the body at a relatively modest pace; fiber slows the absorption of sugar (and other nutrients in our meals) into the body.

WHY *THE ZERO SUGAR DIET* WORKS FOR EVERYONE (AND OTHER PLANS DON'T)

When we talk about keeping blood sugar stable, we often talk about the "glycemic index" (GI) and the "glycemic load" (GL) of foods. Many diets have been built around eating foods with low GI or GL numbers, the better to keep blood sugar spikes at bay. The only problem: New research has shown that these diets may be completely useless.

The glycemic index, or GI, of a certain food is a measure of how quickly its carbohydrates are converted into blood sugar—the higher the number, the faster it causes a blood sugar spike. Glycemic load, on the other hand, looks at both a food's GI and its level of carbohydrates—the idea being that a tablespoon of honey doesn't raise blood sugar as much as a banana, because while the first is made of fast-dissolving fructose, there are far fewer net carbs and overall calories than there are in a full piece of fruit. So while honey has a GI of 55, compared to the banana's 52, the glycemic load of the banana (14) is higher than the glycemic load of the tablespoon of honey (9).

Confused? No wonder: It's pretty tough to have to judge every food based on where it falls on a seemingly random scale. But even if you keep your GL chart handy and only eat foods that fall low on the scale, you might not be doing yourself any favors. The GL scale would rather you eat a container of low-fat yogurt—its GL is 16—than a baked potato, which carries a GL of 28. But

It makes sense, then, that nature paired sugar and fiber together. You see, our current relationship with sugar is codependent and a little unhealthy, sort of like a marriage that still has lots of love, but lots of dysfunction as well. Like a bad boyfriend, sugar is toxic, at least when it's allowed to linger in the bloodstream for too long. So even while we need it to live on, there's also the ever-present threat that it's going to do us harm.

That's why, when sugar hits the bloodstream, the pancreas responds by releasing the hormone insulin. Insulin traffic cops the sugar, help-

---

in reality, the low-fat yogurt has zero fiber and can pack more than 20 grams of added sugars, while the baked potato gives you 7 grams of healthy, belly-filling fiber and no added sugar at all!

New research has shown how misguided this whole GI/GL stuff may be. In a 2015 study, scientists at the Weizmann Institute of Science attached eight hundred people to blood glucose monitors and followed them for a week; over the course of the next seven days, the subjects ate a total of forty-six thousand meals and snacks. The study, published in the journal *Cell,* found that different people responded entirely differently to certain foods; in some, sushi made their blood glucose levels spike, while ice cream caused their levels to rise more slowly. Other subjects had the exact opposite reaction. Blood sugar also rose differently depending on when the food was eaten—for example, right after waking up or right after a workout.

The researchers believe that both lifestyle and the state of one's gut microbiome—basically, the health of the bugs that live in your belly—influence how certain foods affect blood sugar. The researchers were even able to design individualized diets for the participants that helped to keep their blood sugar levels more stable—even though certain "good" foods for one subject might be "bad" foods for another.

So following the GI/GL model, and all those "low GI" diet plans, simply doesn't cut it. *Zero Sugar Diet* is different. It ignores the outdated GI/GL model and focuses instead on using the power of fiber to keep blood sugar levels stable while also feeding your good gut bacteria, providing you with yet another weapon for managing your glucose levels.

ing to convert it into glucose to be stored in the liver and the muscles, and to triglycerides, which are stored in the fat cells.

Back when sugar came with a natural fiber escort, everything was fine. Sugar got released into the bloodstream slowly, thanks to the fiber, and the pancreas could take its measured time doling out the insulin you needed. It was like having your best friend at your back to make sure your loveable but troubled boyfriend didn't get out of hand.

But once we began refining sugar—starting with that first boiled yam—we started delivering sugar more rapidly into our bloodstream. As our craving for sugars grew, so, too, did our technologies; we went from boiled roots to root beer, and started creating foods that dosed us with more rapid-fire sugar than our bodies were designed to handle. These sugars are called "free sugars," meaning anything added to foods by a manufacturer, cook, or consumer, plus sugars that are naturally present in honey, syrups, and fruit juices.

Now worried that this bullying boyfriend called blood sugar is rushing through your system, the pancreas can sometimes overreact, releasing too much insulin and sucking too much sugar out of our blood. That's called hypoglycemia, essentially a sugar crash: that shaky, famished feeling that's different from your standard belly-rumbling hunger. Because our bodies overreacted and stored all that sugar as fat, we suddenly need more sugar, and we need it fast.

So sugar rushes cause us to gain weight in two ways. First, because we can't let sugar linger in the bloodstream, we store it quickly, often in the form of fat. Second, sugar rushes trigger rebound hunger, causing us to go out and find more sugar, and starting the process all over again.

And almost every health fear you've ever stayed up at night worrying about can be linked to this vicious cycle. In a study in *The American Journal of Clinical Nutrition*, researchers looked at thirty-seven different studies on the effects of high-sugar, low-fiber diets and concluded that "higher postprandial glycemia is a universal mechanism for disease progression." In English, that means that "meals that raise your blood sugar will kill you." And not just in one way. If you're susceptible to heart disease, elevated blood sugar will raise your cholesterol levels and your blood pressure. If diabetes runs in your family, it will boost your chances of developing insulin resistance. If obesity is a risk for you, this is the gateway. In fact, this review found links between high-sugar, low-fiber meals and type 2 diabetes, heart disease, stroke, colorectal cancer, and gallbladder disease.

"It's time to reduce our exposure to processed sugar," says Lorenzo Cohen, PhD, of the University of Texas MD Anderson Cancer Center. "We don't need any more research on this." In early 2016, Cohen and

WHAT DOES 100 CALORIES OF ADDED SUGAR LOOK LIKE?

The American Heart Association wants women to take in no more than 100 calories a day of added sugar (150 calories a day for men). But what exactly does that look like?

Each gram of sugar contains 4 calories, so any packaged food with 25 grams of sugar means you've hit your daily limit. To show you exactly how easy it is to hit your sugar limit, here's a snapshot of what 100 calories of added sugar looks like.

½ cup Talente Double Dark Chocolate Gelato

½ cup Ben & Jerry's Peanut Butter Cup ice cream

7 Tbsp Ken's Steak House Lite Asian Sesame with Ginger & Soy Dressing

1 PowerBar Performance Energy Vanilla Crisp bar

3 Tbsp Maggi Sweet Chili Sauce

3 Tbsp La Choy Teriyaki Marinade and Sauce

1½ cups Prego Veggie Smart Smooth and Simple tomato sauce

8 slices Arnold Whole Grains Health Nut bread

6 Tbsp Heinz Tomato Ketchup

4 Tbsp Kraft Thick 'n Spicy Original Barbecue Sauce

6 oz Dannon Fruit on the Bottom Cherry Yogurt

⅛ Pepperidge Farm Coconut 3-Layer Cake

5 Pepperidge Farm Mint Milano cookies

7 Nabisco Chips Ahoy! Original Chocolate Chip cookies

⅔ bag Sour Patch Kids

his colleague Peiying Yang, PhD, conducted an alarming series of animal studies in which more than half of the rodents they exposed to added sugars developed malignant breast cancer tumors by the time they reached six months of age.

"Our brains have been hijacked since our first birthday party with cupcakes," he says. "We need to move ourselves away from sweets in general. Get off that crack! Stop advertising that orange juice is a part of a healthy breakfast. It's not. Eat an orange; that's part of a healthy breakfast."

Why an orange, but not orange juice? Because research has found a simple answer to the sugar crisis: fiber. Fiber lowers the glycemic index (GI) of foods, meaning the rate at which they're turned into toxic blood sugar. In fact, the very same review discovered that habitual intake of fiber from whole grains reduced the risk of coronary heart disease by 20 to 40 percent, and the risk of diabetes by 20 to 30 percent. (Juice extracts the sugar from fruit but eliminates all the fiber, which is why it's verboten on this plan.)

And "eat more fiber" doesn't mean you're going to be nibbling on rabbit food. Fiber comes from a number of delicious sources: whole grains, vegetables, fruits, beans, and nuts. A plate of bean nachos, a cup of chili, a steak salad, some guacamole and chips are all high-fiber options. Just follow the simple recommendations in this plan to keep your fiber up and your sugar down.

Finding the Golden Ratio

In fact, lowering added sugar and increasing fiber have basically the same impact. In a UCLA study of fifty-four overweight teens, individuals who reduced added sugar intake by the equivalent of one can of soda per day over sixteen weeks showed a reduction in belly fat and an improvement in insulin function. Individuals who increased their fiber intake by the equivalent of ½ cup of beans showed exactly the same results.

So to review, the science is irrefutable that cutting sugar helps flatten your belly:

▶ In a review of sixty-eight (!) clinical trials and studies, New Zealand researchers reported in the *British Medical Journal* that increasing sugar intake meant increasing body weight, while reducing sugar meant reducing body weight.

And the science is irrefutable that increasing fiber also helps flatten your belly:

▶ In a study of 1,114 people over five years, researchers reported that for every 10 grams of soluble fiber people ate, their belly fat accumulation was reduced by nearly 4 percent—even if they did nothing else to lose weight.

Now here's where our medical establishment starts to look a lot like the U.S. Congress. . . .

Imagine a series of studies came out showing that people who wore blue clothes ran much faster than people who wore other colors. And imagine there was a ton of scientific proof showing that people who wore red sneakers became far stronger and quicker than those who wore other types of footwear. You'd expect every coach and sports owner to dress his team in blue uniforms and red cleats, right? And you'd expect every single person in your health club to be dressed kinda like Superman, no?

So why doesn't every doctor in the world tell us to focus on cutting sugar and increasing fiber?

Oddly enough, that's not how science works. Despite the mountains of evidence for reducing sugar, and the piles of proof for increasing fiber, no one has really looked at what happens when you combine the two. As Robert Lustig, pediatric endocrinologist at the University of California, San Francisco, explains, "In science, you want to study one variable at a time."

And that's why we've been missing out on the benefits of *Zero Sugar Diet*—until now. In fact, the calculation is so obvious that when we presented this question to Walter Willett, MD, chair of Nutrition at Harvard School of Public Health, he responded, "I don't think such an analysis has been done, but almost surely the effects would be additive—i.e., it's best to do both."

And that's how you get into the Sweet Spot—not just by lowering sugar but by adding fiber to create a balanced safety zone that always keeps you protected from the damaging effects of sugar. This is the greatest weight-loss secret in the world. And it's hiding in plain sight.

Why We Can't Cut Sugar

"Junk Food Junkie." "Sugar Addict." If Walter White had really been a genius, he wouldn't have cooked up methamphetamine; he would have cooked up sugar.

But while other forms of addiction, from drinking and drugs to gambling and even overeating, have established treatment plans, solving our addiction to sugar—and it is an addiction—is more difficult to manage. The reason: From the moment we try sugar as a young child, our brains are forever rewired to crave it.

To battle our overconsumption of sugar, plenty of weight-loss experts have offered low-sugar diets as an alternative. And in theory, a low-sugar diet is a terrific solution: severely reduce the toxin that's causing all that havoc in your body, and you reduce the risk of everything from heart disease to diabetes to dentures. There's only one problem: In the long run, low-sugar diets don't work.

To figure out why, in 2015 scientists at the Monell Chemical Senses Center, a nonprofit scientific institute that studies taste and smell, put a group of sugary-soda drinkers on a reduced-sugar program, replacing 40 percent of their daily sugar calories with fats, proteins, and complex carbohydrates. A second group of soda drinkers continued with their regular sugar-addled diet. After three months, those on a reduced-sugar diet reported that desserts like vanilla pudding tasted very sweet, while the control group rated the same foods as less sweet.

Ideally, that would have meant that after three months on a low-sugar diet, the test subjects would have lost their desire for sweets.

But unfortunately, the low-sugar group didn't get turned off by the overly sweet taste. In fact, they reported enjoying it just as much as the high-sugar group. And once the restriction period ended, the low-sugar group quickly reverted to their previous high-sugar diets.

If you love sugar—and you love sugar, don't even try to deny it—then breaking your desire for it may not be possible. But what is possible is to reduce sugar's impact on your body, and to protect yourself from its consequences while stripping away unwanted pounds, by finding your Sweet Spot. That's the unique premise of *Zero Sugar Diet*.

DOUGHNUTS FOR DINNER

A Glazed Donut from Dunkin' is 260 calories, with 1 gram of fiber and 12 grams of sugar. So there won't be any doughnuts on your menu for the next 14 days.

But while you know that doughnuts are sugar festivals, you won't believe what other foods have as much sugar as a Glazed Donut, or more.

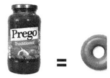

Prego Heart Smart Traditional Italian Sauce, ¾ cup: **¾ donut**

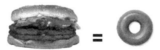

Burger King Double Whopper: **1 donut**

Hunt's Tomato Ketchup, 3 Tablespoons: **1 donut**

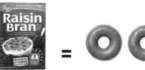

Raisin Bran, serving: **1½ donuts**

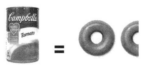

Campbell's Creamy Tomato Soup, 1 cup: **1½ donuts**

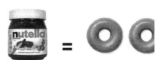

Nutella, 2 Tbsp: **1¾ donuts**

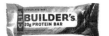 =

Clif Builder's Protein Bar, Chocolate Mint: **1¾ donuts**

 =

Dannon Fruit on the Bottom, Blueberry: **2 donuts**

 =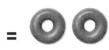

Hungry Man Dinner, Roasted Turkey: **2 donuts**

 =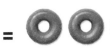

McDonald's Fruit & Maple Oatmeal: **2⅓ donuts**

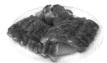 =

Chili's Dr. Pepper BBQ Ribs (full): **2⅓ donuts**

 =

Coca Cola, 1 can: **3½ donuts**

 =

Applebee's Oriental Grilled Chicken Salad: **4½ donuts**

 =

Dunkin' Donuts Coffee Coolatta with Cream: **5½ donuts**

EXCUSES, EXCUSES

I Reached Out to Scores of Food Marketers to Find Out Why Their Products Were So Loaded with Sugar. Few, If Any, Had a Good Answer.

In life, we all understand that risky behaviors come freighted with potential consequences. If you buy yourself a motorcycle, you know you're upping your chances of becoming street pizza. If you take up hang gliding, you accept that there's a good possibility you might hit a wall—literally. And if you go out clubbing with Miley Cyrus, it's nobody's fault but your own if you wake up with a piercing some-place weird. That's the cost of signing up—and that's okay, as long as we go into it with eyes wide open (and perhaps a signed waiver).

It ought to be that way with our food choices, as well. We all know that Baskin-Robbins isn't a health-food store, that eating too much birthday cake can cut down on your future birthdays, and that trick-or-treat will rot your teeth. When we're faced with such indulgences, we understand that it's up to us to eat in moderation, or bear the consequences.

But what about companies that produce foods we think of as "healthy," or at least not harmful—foods that we might eat every day without ever suspecting that they come packed with sugar? Why does Sunbelt Bakery slip 16 grams of sugar into its healthy-sounding Fruit & Grain Bars? Why does a single tablespoon of Hunt's Ketchup contain a full teaspoon (4 grams) of sugar? Why are there 7 grams of sugar in a Lean Cuisine Mushroom Mezzaluna Ravioli (and why does sugar appear three times, and glucose once, in its ingredients list)?

And that's not even taking into consideration what's happening at restaurants like Red Robin. We expect their sundaes to be loaded with unhealthy ingredients, but why do they offer a fourteen-piece Boneless Bar Wings with Banzai Sauce with 47 grams of sugar (that's a teaspoon of sugar per wing!)? Why does a family-size order of Sonic Onion Rings come with 51 grams of sugar, when you could get three orders of the same food at Applebee's and still get only half the sugar? Not that Applebee's gets a free pass: Order your child a Kid's Chocolate Shake and you're serving your little one 88 grams of sugar—nearly double what an adult woman should have in a day!

As I've said throughout this book, it's not the occasional desserts that are taking the biggest toll on our bodies; it's the everyday hits of sugar that we don't even realize we're getting. And when we do indulge, we often get far more sugar from our sweets than we might normally expect.

To figure out what the heck is going on here, I decided to reach out to the food manufacturers themselves, and launched a letter-writing inquiry aimed at forty popular brands. I asked them, Why does your product include so much sugar, when comparable products on the market are made successfully with less? For example, why does Golden Island Beef Jerky contain 11 grams of sugar per serving, when a similar product from Brooklyn Biltong contains zero? Why does Quaker sell a granola (its Natural Granola Oats, Honey, Raisins & Almonds) with 13 grams of sugar per half cup, when a tiny company like Engine 2 Plant-Strong can sell a Plain Jane Granola with just 7 grams in the same size serving? And what's up with the sugar and molasses in your peanut butter, Jif? Smucker's doesn't need added sugar. (Shouldn't it be called Jif Creamy Peanut-and-Sugar Butter?)

I'd love to report that America's food purveyors were eager to join me in examining the use of sugar in their products. But mostly, they seemed interested in how far into the sand they could dig their heads. Of the forty queries I sent out, each followed up with phone calls, fewer than one in three responded. In fact, the reaction from the food industry could be categorized like this:

"Yikes, this sugar question is scary. We are going to ignore you and hope that it goes away."   60 percent

Olive Garden, Jif, Nutella Global, Ghirardelli, Dunkin' Donuts, and Red Robin were among the companies that didn't respond to our repeated requests for comment.

"We offer a variety of foods and flavors for all tastes, so it's really your fault if you buy our sugary products."

17.5 percent

From giant purveyors of nominally healthy foods such as Quaker Oats to small "health food" companies such as Angie's BOOMCHICKAPOP to fast-food joints not known for healthy eating, the most often heard excuse was, "You could always buy one of our other products." It's a great argument for why added sugars should be displayed as prominently as calories; two foods of equal calories don't have the same impact on your health when one of them is loaded with sugar.

Sample quote: *"We recognize our customers may come to us for a variety of reasons and occasions. That's why our menu offers a variety of choices—including more indulgent treats to an ever-expanding array of more wholesome options."* **—McDonald's**

"We're just giving the people what they want."

10 percent

In the case of foods in which sugar is not part of the food's traditional recipe, most responses boiled down to, "That's the American public's preferred flavor." This despite the fact that people the world over have been enjoying soup, tomato sauce, and other recipes without added sugar for centuries.

Sample quote: *"We also add sugar to offset the acidic, or tart, taste tomatoes can sometimes have, and balance the flavors."* **—Campbell's Soup**

"We hear you, and we're trying."

7.5 percent

Pizza Hut, Nestlé, and Kellogg's are among the companies that responded by acknowledging that sugar was a concern, and pointing out that they've already taken steps to reduce sugar. (Nesquik's most popular chocolate powder now contains 35 percent less sugar than it did in 2000, while Pizza Hut said it was in the process of eliminating their most sugary chicken wings—its Wingstreet Bone-Out Wings in Sweet Chili with BBQ Wing Sauce carried a ridiculous 11 grams of sugar per wing—and replacing it with a sauce with just 1 gram of sugar per wing.)

Sample quote: *"The majority of our cereals now have 10 g or less of sugar per 30 g serving, and by 2020, 90 percent of our Kellogg's cereals will have 10 g of sugar or less."*

Kellogg's also pointed out that they've already reduced the sugar in Frosted Flakes, Froot Loops, and Apple Jacks.

To those companies that refuse to address the sugar content of their foods—and to companies like Starbucks, Long John Silver's, and Cheesecake Factory that either obscure their nutritional information or refuse to list the amount of sugar appearing in their foods on their nutritional charts—it's time to step up and do a better job of protecting the people who are putting their hard-earned money into your pockets. And to that handful of companies willing to face the issue head-on, I say kudos—and I'll be watching to make sure you keep your promises.

"Here's some health mumbo-jumbo we can throw at you so you'll stop talking about this sugar thing." 2.5 percent

Despite pointed questions about the amount of sugar in specific products, some companies preferred to fall back on their existing health halo, ignoring what has become more and more obvious: Sugar is bad for you, even if it's sourced from organic soil fertilized with the sacrificial blood of Andean virgins.

Sample quote: *"[W]e over the past year have been working to transition our granola products to be gluten-free. This transition is in response to the request from our customers to offer more gluten-free options. We've also made a goal to obtain non-GMO product verification and/or USDA organic certification. . . ."*
—**Back to Nature Foods Company**

THE SUGARIEST FOODS IN AMERICA

Meet the Twenty-five with More Sugar than You Should Eat in an Entire Day

Even the U.S. government thinks you're sweet enough.

In fact, for the first time ever, the USDA has issued guidelines recommending that Americans keep their consumption of added sugars low—to no more than 10 percent of overall calories, or about 180 calories a day for women and 200 for men.

That means 45 grams of sugar a day, tops, or about eleven teaspoons. But organizations from the American Heart Association to the World Health Organization recommend cutting that number further; they say no more than 25 grams of added sugar a day (about six sugar packets) is best for optimal health.

But let's go easy on ourselves; let's pretend for once that the government actually does know best, and that eleven teaspoons of sugar a day is A-OK. Still, you'll be surprised how easy it is to eat that much; in fact, the average American woman consumes about twenty-five teaspoons of sugar a day, or about 125 pieces of Jelly Belly a day.

But if you're not popping jelly beans or chugging high-fructose corn syrup, where are all those sugar calories coming from? Surprisingly, a lot come from foods you'd never think of as "sugary." Here's our list of twenty-five surprising foods with more sugar than the USDA allows, ranked from crazy bad to *insanely* bad.

25/Smucker's Blueberry Syrup (¼ cup)

200 calories | 0 g fat | 51 g carbs | 0 g fiber | **44 g sugar** | 0 g protein

If you thought for a moment that blueberry syrup was healthier than the standard variety, disabuse yourself of that notion now. This serving size is for a mere ¼ cup, but unless you're using a measuring spoon, you're almost definitely overserving yourself—and blowing through your daily sugar allotment.

24/Dunkin' Donuts Blueberry Muffin

460 calories | 15 g fat (3 g saturated) | 76 g carbs | 2 g fiber
44 g sugar | 6 g protein

You thought you were making the healthy choice by opting for the fruit muffin instead of the doughnut at Dunkin', but you could have had four Apple n Spice Donuts and still not eaten as much sugar. Add a small latte with almond milk and you're up to **57 g of sugar** to start your morning—and most likely crash your afternoon.

23/Red Robin Boneless Bar Wing 'N' Yukon Chips (with Banzai Sauce)

1,263 calories | 56 g fat | 141 g carbs | 19 g fiber | **47 g sugar** | 56 g protein

At Red Robin, "Banzai" is code for "sugar." The same meal with Buzzard Sauce has just 1 gram of sugar.

22/Applebee's Grilled Shrimp 'N Spinach Salad

1,000 calories | 66 g fat (10 g saturated) | 67 g carbs | 12 g fiber
50 g sugar | 44 g protein

Eating this food is like getting caught speeding on a road with no posted speed limit signs. Everything sure looks free and clear, and just check out those health words: Grilled! Spinach! Salad! A great example of how sugar sneaks up on us even when we think we're eating healthy.

21/Sonic Handmade Onion Rings (Family Size)

1,610 calories | 79 g fat (14 g saturated, 1.5 g trans) | 202 g carbs
10 g fiber | **51 g sugar** | 23 g protein

Okay, it is "family size," so for sure you'll be sharing. But even if you're a family of four, you're still getting as much sugar from a small portion of rings as you'd get from a Little Debbie Doughnut Stick.

20/Applebee's Sweet Potato Fries & Dips

1,070 calories | 64 g fat (13 g saturated, 1 g trans) | 118 g carbs | 7 g fiber
51 g sugar | 7 g protein

Sweet potatoes are already naturally sweet (hence the name), but many restaurants feel the need to guild the lily, sugar-wise.

19/Sonic Blackberry Green Iced Tea (Large)

210 calories | 0 g fat | 55 g carbs | 0 g fiber | **55 g sugar** | 0 g protein

We've touted the health benefits of green tea enough that you must surely think it's always a great choice, but at Sonic, somebody's cooking up a concoction that turns this healthy drink on its head.

18/Chili's Crispy Honey Chipotle Crispers with BBQ Sauce

1,410 calories | 51 g fat (9 g saturated) | 189 g carbs | 9 g fiber
63 g sugar | 56 g protein

With the word "crisp" in the title twice, you'd think fat would be your biggest worry, but Chili's manages to pack 52 grams of sugar into the actual Crisper itself—before even adding on the BBQ Sauce.

17/Olive Garden Strawberry Smoothie

330 calories | 1 g fat (0.5 g saturated) | 74 g carbs | 0 g fiber
65 g sugar | 5 g protein

If you thought you were doing the healthy thing by ordering the berry smoothie and skipping the cocktail, you're in for a surprise. Devoid of fiber, this fruity drink has nearly twice as much sugar as a Sprite.

16/Pizza Hut Wingstreet Bone-Out Wings in Sweet Chili (6) with
3 Ounces of BBQ Wing Sauce

830 calories | 27 g fat (4.5 g saturated) | 2,490 mg sodium | 112 g carbs
4 g fiber | **68 g sugar** | 31 g protein

The culprit here isn't the bird itself, but Pizza Hut's Sweet Chili sauce—which is really just a fancy name for a viscous pool of brown sugar. Next time a craving strikes, keep your diabetes risk in check by ordering the Naked wings, and enjoy six of 'em. This simple, slimming swap will save you 39 grams of sugar—the equivalent of seven rolls of Smarties.

15/Chili's Caribbean Salad with Grilled Chicken

720 calories | 28 g fat (4.5 g saturated) | 1,170 mg sodium
86 g carbs | 9 g fiber | **69 g sugar** | 36 g protein

A salad with grilled chicken—every skinny girl's cliché lunch, right? But this is a terrible example of sugar hiding in a seemingly healthful dish. After eating Chili's Caribbean Salad—and its 9 doughnuts' worth of sugar—you'll be less bikini-confident than ever. Order the zesty Southwest Chicken Soup with a side salad instead. You'll save 60 grams of the sweet stuff, and be swimsuit ready by summer.

14/Friendly's Honey BBQ Chicken Strips

1,580 calories | 82 g fat (15 g saturated) | 3,170 mg sodium
168 g carbs | 5 g fiber | **73 g sugar** | 43 g protein

These Chicken Strips are distinctly un-Friendly, thanks to a Honey BBQ sauce that could put your dentists' kids through private school. Choose the Turkey Tips—bite-size pieces of protein-packed grilled meat—and save 1,020 calories and 68 grams of sugar!

13/P.F. Chang's Sesame Chicken

890 calories | 35 g fat (6 g saturated) | 2,250 mg sodium | 82 g carbs
6 g fiber | **76 g sugar** | 66 g protein

Duck! Your dinner table is about to get ransacked by the Stay Puft Marsh-mallow Man. Covered in a thick coating of sauce, Sesame Chicken has never looked like the healthiest pick on the menu, but you probably didn't sus-pect that it has as much sugar as twenty jumbo marshmallows! Stay away from this dish, and the Sweet & Sour Chicken, too—that one came in a close second with a whopping 69 grams of sugar (but at least it has the word "sweet" in the name). Instead, ask your server to bring you the Dynamite Shrimp starter with a small side of Spinach with Garlic as your entrée. You'll get that sweet, tangy taste you crave for a fraction of the calories and sugar.

12/California Pizza Kitchen Full Moroccan-Spiced Chicken Salad

1,500 calories | 99 g fat (10 g saturated) | 1,380 mg sodium
128 g carbs | 27 g fiber | **80 g sugar** | 43 g protein

I'm pretty sure Morocco will be annoyed to learn their top spice, according to CPK, is sugar. For something that looks and tastes similar, but saves you 68 grams of sugar, ask for the Roast Veggie and Grilled Chicken salad. Ask for the dressing on the side and only use a few spoonfuls.

11/Applebee's Kid's Chocolate Shake

820 calories | 35 g fat (20 g saturated) | 110 g carbs | 2 g fiber
88 g sugar | 19 g protein

Okay, we know chocolate shakes aren't healthy. But this is a child's drink with as much sugar as an adult should have in two whole days.

10/Applebee's Riblets Platter with Honey BBQ Sauce

1,100 calories | 51 g fat (17 g saturated) | 104 g carbs | 4 g fiber
92 g sugar | 68 g protein

Yes, honey is an added sugar, no matter what Winnie the Pooh says. In fact, 82 grams of the sugar in this platter comes from the sauce.

9/Jamba Juice Acai Primo Bowl (24 Ounces)

740 calories | 15 g fat (4 g saturated) | 148 g carbs | 16 g fiber
96 g sugar | 12 g protein

"Energy bowls" are a new trend at juice places, but remember that another word for "energy" is "calories." While some of the sugar comes from fruit, much of it comes from honey and granola, leading to more than two days' worth of sweetness.

8/Cheesecake Factory Teriyaki Chicken

1,320 calories | 19 g fat (3 g saturated) | 3,993 mg sodium | 207 g carbs
2 g fiber | **96 g sugar** | 70 g protein

"Terror-yaki" is more like it. This entrée—which could only have been
conceived in a "factory"—is the sugar equivalent of 3.5 Snickers Bars,
and comes topped with two days' worth of salt. As much as we hate the
idea of ordering anything called "Skinnylicious" in front of a dinner date,
at Cheesecake Factory that might be your best bet.

7/Red Lobster Alotta Colada

580 calories | 7 g fat (7 g saturated) | 109 g carbs | 7 g fiber
98 g sugar | 2 g protein

Like chugging three cans of Coke in one sitting. Alotta Colada
means alotta you, too. Just one of these drinks before dinner gives
you more than two days' worth of sugars. We know alcoholic
drinks aren't a health food, but consider that a Long Island Iced Tea
contains just 15 grams of sugar.

6/Panda Express 2-entrée plate with Chow Mein, SweetFire Chicken Breast, and Beijing Beef

2,310 calories | 107 g fat (19 g saturated) | 2,840 mg sodium
230 g carbs | 11 g fiber | **100 g sugar** | 68 g protein

This is the sugar equivalent of eight McDonald's Baked Hot Apple
Pies! "Panda Express" accurately describes both what you're going
to look like and how long it's going to take you to get there.
They call them "SweetFire" meats for a reason. Listen to the warning
shot, and take evasive action.

5/Perkins Berry Blueberry Pancakes with 2 Ounces Syrup

1,000 calories | 24 g fat (9 g saturated) | 975 mg sodium
180 g carbs | 7 g fiber | **105 g sugar** | 15 g protein

Okay, you know pancakes with syrup is gonna be sugary. But holy cow,
Perkins, how did you manage to pack two days' worth of sugar into one
breakfast? This is the sugar equivalent of four Dairy Queen Vanilla Cones!

4/Jamba Juice Strawberry Surf Rider (28 Ounces)

590 calories | 2 g fat (1 g saturated) | 142 g carbs | 4 g fiber
128 g sugar | 4 g protein

Strawberry Couch Rider might be a better name for this sugary combination
of fruit, lime sherbet, and lemonade. Even downgrading to the smallest size,
16 ounces, will still put you at 70 grams of sweet stuff.

3/Cheesecake Factory French Toast Napoleon with Syrup

2,880 calories | 190 g fat (95 g saturated) | 1,585 mg sodium | 160 g carbs
7 g fiber | **139 g sugar** | 29 g protein

French Toast Napoleon, meet your Waterloo. This one breakfast
will feed you nearly three days' worth of sugar, a day and a half's worth
of calories, and nearly a week's worth of saturated fat. Oh, and
somehow they squeezed a full day of sodium onto the plate as well.
In this war of European powers, we'll take the English muffin over
the French toast any day.

2/Boston Market St. Louis Style BBQ Ribs Half-Rack with Cinnamon Apples and Sweet Potato Casserole

1,860 calories | 90 g fat (33 g saturated) | 3,620 mg sodium
201 g carbs | 10 g fiber | **162 g sugar** | 68 g protein

With a holiday weekend's worth of sugar and two days of sodium,
your blood sugar and blood pressure will be in a race to see who can
redline faster. Opting for the Quarter Skinless Rotisserie Chicken
plate will save you a whopping 144 grams of sugar—enough that you
can enjoy what you really want: dessert.

1/Smoothie King The Hulk Strawberry

1,928 calories | 64 g fat (26 g saturated) | 290 g carbs | 16 g fiber
250 g sugar | 50 g protein

"Blended to help you get toned, build muscle, last longer or recover faster"
is the claim Smoothie King makes for its line of Fitness Blends, of which
The Hulk is the beefiest. It contains butter pecan ice cream and a proprietary
"weight gain blend." We're pretty sure we know what's in that: about
five days' worth of sugar.

Special Report

WHY FIBER IS THE PERFECT SOLUTION, AND HOW TO MAKE IT WORK FOR YOU

THERE'S NOTHING SEXY ABOUT FIBER.

Fiber is like the NPR of nutrition. It's there, we know it's good for us, but . . . meh. Who wants to focus on educational radio when there's always a new Beyoncé track dropping? And who wants to focus on fiber when it's so much more fun trying to figure out when the next McRib will be released?

So chances are you haven't thought much about fiber, where it comes from, or what it does once it's inside of you. Our grandparents called fiber "roughage," but let's face it—they were tougher than we are. And that term doesn't really tell the story of what this critical, lifesaving nutrient does.

Fiber is a type of carbohydrate that makes up the structural material in the leaves, stems, and roots of vegetables, grains, and fruits. It's like the spine of plants. But unlike sugar and starch—two other types of carbs—fiber stays intact until it nears the end of your digestive tract. This is what makes fiber beneficial.

There are two basic types of fiber, and they have separate functions.

▶ **Insoluble fiber** is found in wheat bran, nuts, and many vegetables. Its structure is thick and rough, and it won't dissolve in water, so it zips through your digestive tract and increases the bulk of your stool. (Definitely nothing sexy here.)

▶ **Soluble fiber** is found in oats, beans, barley, and some fruits. It dissolves in water to form a gel-like material in your digestive tract. This allows it to slow the absorption of sugar into your bloodstream. What's more, soluble fiber, when eaten regularly, has been shown to slightly lower LDL (bad) cholesterol levels.

The ironic thing is that fiber is essentially a bundle of sugar molecules. Digestion is what happens when the enzymes in your body break apart the bonds that hold food molecules together, but fiber molecules are held together by chemical bonds that your body has trouble breaking. In fact, your stomach and small intestine are powerless against fiber. It's not until it all lands way down at the bottom of your digestive tract, at your large intestine, that soluble fiber gets converted to short-chain fatty acids, which do provide a few calories. A gram of regular carbohydrates has about 4 calories, as does a gram of soluble fiber, according to the FDA. (Insoluble fiber has essentially zero calories, because even the large intestine can't break it down, and it just . . . moves along.)

In Stone Age times, man may have eaten as much as 100 grams of fiber a day, but modern food processing has reduced that total to about 15 grams a day. And thanks to that fiber shortage, here's what we're now missing:

Fiber prevents your body from experiencing a sugar rush.

Think of a time-release medicine capsule. You know, the ones that come in bullet-shaped capsules that look like oblong plastic beads. In a time-release medication, the active ingredients are encased in an indigestible polymer container; as the capsule makes its way down the fantastic voyage of your digestive tract, the medicine slowly works its way out, into your system, so your body gets a continuous dose over several hours.

This is exactly what fiber does to sugar. Soluble fiber—think of the inside of an apple—forms a gel-like paste once it hits your digestive system. (If you eat oatmeal, you have an idea of what this gummy paste might look like.) While this paste slows the progress of food down your pipes, keeping you feeling fuller longer, it also prevents the quick absorption of sugar molecules, which are trapped within the paste just like the medicine trapped inside your time-release capsule.

(To maximize this effect, however, you need to stay properly hydrated. You can drink your six to eight glasses a day like every Web story or magazine article you've ever read tells you to,

or you can do one better and read your body's own signals: If you pee clear, you're in the clear. If you pee yella, you need some more water, fella.)

"The goal of reducing added sugars and increasing fiber is to reduce the hit on the liver," explains Dr. Lustig of the University of California, San Francisco. "Increasing the fiber forms a gel on the inside of the intestine, which delays absorption, and makes more of it go through the intestine where the bacteria will chew it up instead of it going to your liver."

Fiber feeds the bacteria in your colon, starting a chemical reaction that flips off your appetite switch.

Your belly has a posse.

Way, way down at the very end of your digestive tract—past the long drop of your esophagus, beyond the acidic stew of your stomach, and far beyond the twenty-three-foot labyrinthine length of your small intestine— there's a SWAT team of killers ready to do whatever it takes to keep you slim.

These creatures are your gut bacteria. And while your digestive system—heck, your whole body—is really just one giant infestation of more than eighty trillion different microbes, when it comes to your weight, the buggers at the bottom of your digestive tract, chilling in your colon, are the ones that control a series of master switches. When you deliver food to them, they deliver something back to you: weight loss.

In fact, while scientists have long known that eating fiber helps us control hunger, they didn't really understand why until 2014, when researchers at the Imperial College of London discovered an anti-appetite molecule called acetate. This molecule is released naturally when our SWAT team digests fiber. During the digestion process, the fiber ferments and releases a large amount of acetate as a waste product. Once created, the acetate travels from the colon to the liver and the heart, and eventually winds up in the hypothalamus, the region of the brain that controls hunger. Once there, it causes the firing of specialized neurons that signal us to stop eating.

Fiber prevents fat from forming inside your belly.

Pity your poor liver. It gets none of the glamor or attention of your stomach, and nobody ever checks in on it the way they do your colon. And the things you've put it through! (Remember those off-campus happy hours?)

But unless you're a serious drinker, your liver isn't getting beaten up by the couple of glasses of merlot you down at night. It's getting beaten up by the sugar in your diet. In fact, many of us have unhealthy levels of fat accumulating around our liver and pancreas due to the effects of the high doses of fructose we eat, according to a report in *Current Opinion in Clinical Nutrition & Metabolic Care*. Sugar does the same thing to your liver that shots of bourbon do; a recent study at the Mayo Clinic found that one in ten cases of liver failure is now caused by nonalcoholic steatohepatitis, or NASH. (Studies show that Hispanics in particular are at elevated risk for liver fat accumulation triggered by sugar because of a higher frequency of genes that predispose them for fatty liver.)

Because the liver stores sugar for later use, when it gets overwhelmed, it does the only thing it can to off-load the extra calories; it creates fat cells in which to store the excess energy. But these cells are actually toxic to the liver in the long run; these types of fat cells, called visceral fat (because they're up against your innards), release a variety of compounds collectively called adipokines. They're a murderer's row of troublemakers, including resistin, a hormone that undermines your body's ability to metabolize glucose and leads to diabetes, and tumor necrosis factor, which is just as bad as it sounds—it causes inflammatory issues including psoriasis, Crohn's disease, and various forms of arthritis.

The pancreas, too, starts to grow a layer of unhealthy fat. In fact, type 2 diabetes may be caused in part by fat accumulating in the pancreas, according to a 2015 British study. In the study, total body weight loss that results in just 1 gram of fat being drained from the pancreas is enough to allow this insulin-producing organ to return to normal functioning and to reverse diabetes in people suffering from it.

But simply boosting fiber intake can reduce the damage to our liver and pancreas and give these poor, battered organs a chance to step up and clear out our systems. In a pilot study done in Portugal, subjects with nonalcoholic fatty liver disease received 10 grams a day of soluble fiber for three months. One hundred percent of the subjects showed a reduction in body mass index, waist circumference, and insulin resistance. Two-thirds showed lowered cholesterol levels and 75 percent showed normal liver enzymes.

Fiber lets us eat meat and other fatty fare without increasing our risk of heart attack or stroke.

In a study in the journal *Lipids*, researchers compared men who

Fiber, or Fibber?

Fiber is showing up in everything these days, especially things that shouldn't have fiber, like yogurt, grape juice, and even artificial sweeteners. If this seems impossible, remember that fiber in the end is really just a type of sugar molecule; you don't have to see, feel, or taste fiber for it to be present. And when you see foods touting fiber where it doesn't belong —Activia yogurt, for example—what you're really seeing is something called "functional" fiber, meaning that it's created and added to processed foods.

Functional fibers can be made from actual plants, or they can be created from bacteria or yeast; as long as this new creation can be shown to do at least one of the things that natural fiber can do, like provide food for your gut bacteria or increase stool weight, manufacturers can label it as fiber.

But these Frankenfibers don't necessarily provide you with the same benefits as naturally occurring fiber. Inulin, for example, a soluble fiber extracted from the chicory root (and used in Activia) is, indeed, a prebiotic, which means it promotes the growth of healthy bacteria in the gut. But it doesn't have the same cholesterol-lowering effect as the fiber found in oat bran. (And worse, Activia's ingredients label lists both fructose and sugar before fruit or inulin, which is why this "fiber-rich" yogurt still has 16 grams of sugar to just 3 grams of fiber.)

Other artificial fibers are made from sugar, like polydextrose and maltodextrin (in particular "resistant maltodextrin," which goes through a special process to make it indigestible). While these additives do indeed bulk up the foods without adding calories, they haven't been shown to have any impact on regularity or any aspect of digestive health. Bottom line: If you can't figure out WHY this food has fiber, it probably doesn't have the kind of fiber you want.

ate a "healthy American diet" to those who ate the same diet, but supplemented with fiber from legumes. (That's anything that grows in a pod, like peanuts, beans, lentils, or those giant cockroaches from *Alien*.) They found that the high-fiber, high-legume diet improved serum lipid profiles in men compared to a healthy diet with less fiber.

One of the reasons why is that soluble fiber, during its long, slow descent down the digestive tract, binds to bile acids in the intestines. Bile is like the dishwasher gel of the body: It breaks up the oil you've eaten. It's the liver's job to make bile acids, and guess what it makes them from? Cholesterol. When fiber hijacks these acids and strips them out of your digestive system, it's like you've turned on the dishwasher's rinse cycle. All the bile goes down the drain, and the liver has to pull out the Dyson and suck cholesterol out of your bloodstream in order to make more.

But if you eat a meal without fiber, the bile isn't stripped away. It's simply reabsorbed into the body, along with all the toxins and fats that it helped to digest.

It's like you stopped the wash cycle before it got to "rinse." Now your liver has to do the work of scrubbing the broken-down food particles out of your system, instead of getting a fresh, clean start. And since it can just recycle the bile it's reabsorbed, it will leave your cholesterol alone, so it can accumulate in your bloodstream.

Sugar has a much different effect than fiber. Sugar is metabolized in the liver—adding to the organ's workload—and increases levels of triglycerides.

Fiber stimulates our satisfaction and sleep hormones.

Studies show that a fiber-rich meal stimulates the release of a hormone called CCK. Sounds like a new fragrance from Calvin Klein, but it's actually short for cholecystokinin, and it works within our bodies to help us feel satiated by slowing the flow of food through our bodies. It also regulates sleep, so if you feel satisfied and sleepy after a meal, you have CCK to thank. And who doesn't want to fall asleep with a smile on her face?

**Fiber allows us
the maximum amount
of dietary flexibility—
no more restrictions!**

It doesn't matter where your fiber intake comes from, as long as it comes from natural foods. (There's that flexibility factor again!) In a study at the University of South Carolina, subjects who ate an average of 16.6 grams of fiber per day were put on one of two diets that increased their fiber intake to an average of 28.4 grams a day. One group got their additional fiber primarily from beans, while the second got theirs from fruits, vegetables, and whole grains. After four weeks, both groups had lost the same amount of weight—an average of three pounds each—and both groups reported less hunger and more satiety. This despite the fact that the subjects didn't exercise or take any other steps toward weight loss other than to boost their fiber.

chapter 5

WHAT TO EXPECT ON THE ZERO SUGAR DIET

Our test panelists walk you through their amazing, life-changing results

LESS FAT. LESS HUNGER. More energy. More muscle. And best of all, a flat, lean belly.

For many of us, these goals seem out of reach, like dreams from a more innocent time that has long since passed us by. But for the more than eleven hundred men and women who joined the Zero Sugar Test Panel, they're not dreams any longer. In just fourteen days, these panelists turned their long-deferred hopes into reality.

For Donna Scott, fifty-two, a field technician from Las Cruces, New Mexico, weight loss always seemed like a slow, onerous task, one that involved hunger, sacrifice, and more discipline than any of us would want to muster. Yet on *Zero Sugar Diet*, Scott's extra weight seemed simply to fall off of her—a remarkable 15 pounds gone in only fourteen days. From a starting weight of 175 pounds, she is now a lean, mean 160.

And it's not just the amount of fat our test panelists lost, it's the type of fat: dangerous, unsightly belly fat. "My waist has gone down in size, and I feel healthier!" she says.

"In addition to losing 11.2 pounds, I also lost one inch off my waist," echoes David Menkhaus, sixty-two, of Liberty Township, Ohio.

"My belly is flatter and people are noticing!" says Sandy Villegas, a retired teacher from Monroe Township, New Jersey. "I have had very few cravings and am eating much less than before." More important, after just a few weeks, Sandy's doctor decided to take her off her blood pressure medication.

And that has been, for me, the most exciting aspect of *Zero Sugar Diet*: its potential to save people's lives by reducing their risk of heart disease, diabetes, stroke, and cancer. And fast. Sure, flattening your belly may have the biggest impact on how people see you: After all, it's the very first part of you to arrive anywhere you travel. But we know for certain that it has the biggest impact on your health.

Once you cut out added sugars and add fiber, you dramatically reduce the impact of food on your liver, relieving that beleaguered organ of its fat-storing duties and allowing it to do what it does best: manage your cholesterol levels. That's why I urge you to see a doctor before and after your fourteen-day journey, to prove to yourself how powerful this program can be. "About ten days in my doctor did blood work, and the results were fantastic!" says Wanda Tapp of Little Rock, Arkansas. "Cholesterol, etc., were better than they had ever been."

Meanwhile, in Albuquerque, New Mexico, disabled Army veteran Richard Casados had been fighting to get his weight and blood pressure down ever since an injury put an end to his running program. In fact, he'd set a goal to get his weight down from 160 to a more comfortable 154 over the course of two months. "Then this Zero Sugar test came along," he says. In just a couple of weeks he had already lost 4 pounds, and decided to set a more ambitious weight-loss goal of 148. But more important, Casados had been closely monitoring his own health. His blood pressure and pulse rate had both dropped, his blood glucose levels were stable, and his body fat—already a healthy 21.8 percent—dropped down to 20.2 percent. "This *Zero Sugar Diet* really works!" he says.

And best of all, it works for everyone. Every one of the members of the test panel who completed the program reported to me that they lost weight, and many of them lost between ten and fifteen pounds in just fourteen days.

Dropping Pounds— and Changing Lives—Fast

Wait a minute: Fifteen pounds in fourteen days? Isn't that too much?

Perhaps you've been told that rapid weight loss isn't healthy, or that it will lead to yo-yo dieting, or that the results won't "stick." Dropping ten to fifteen pounds in just two weeks not only seems like a stretch, it sounds downright bad for you, especially in our culture, where "all things in moderation" is the catchall response to any over-the-top challenge. You have to lose weight slowly if you want to keep it off in the long term, right?

Wrong. Research consistently shows that rapid weight loss, the kind experienced by the Zero Sugar Test Panel, is exactly what leads to long-term success. In fact, a recent review of literature by researchers at Copenhagen University's Department of Nutrition, Exercise, and Sports found that whether you're looking at diets, workout plans, or even drug therapies, those who drop the most pounds in the first two weeks or so are also the most likely to have lost the most weight two years later. In fact, you're five times as likely to succeed in your long-term weight-loss goals if you start out of the gate by dropping pounds rapidly, according to a 2013 study in the *International Journal of Behavioral Medicine.*

And that's exactly what *Zero Sugar Diet* is designed to do—regardless of your age or your lifestyle. Consider forty-five-year-old Ray Micknowski of Pittsburgh, Pennsylvania. A medical biller, he's pretty much tied to a desk all day. Yet without taking on an intense exercise program, and without restricting calories, he dropped a pound a day on the fourteen-day plan. Isela Estrada, a thirty-four-year-old sales administrator from Tucson, Arizona, weighed more than three hundred pounds when she took the fourteen-day challenge, and stripped off nearly eleven pounds in two weeks. And Andy Turner, a nurse's aide in Dorset, England, dropped more than ten pounds in fourteen days.

Expand the Mind, Shrink the Belly

But this plan doesn't just put your body on autopilot. It gives you the skills to manage your own weight for decades to come. Indeed, many test panelists told us that their experience on *Zero Sugar Diet* helped them become more attuned to what they were eating. "I am more consistent with reading food labels, which I have not done in the past," says LaShawn Jones, forty-four, of Harrisburg, Pennsylvania.

And that alone is an enormous leap forward. Becoming more aware—not just of what you eat, but of every aspect of your daily life—can have a serious impact on your body and your overall health. In a 2015 study, Brown University researchers asked nearly four hundred people to complete a mindfulness awareness survey, which asked whether subjects agreed with such questions as "I find it difficult to stay focused on what's happening in the present." Then, they X-rayed the subjects' bellies to determine their degree of belly fat. What they found was that the higher people scored on the mindfulness survey, the less visceral fat they were likely to have. People who are less mind-

FOODS THAT FIGHT SUGAR CRAVINGS

If you find yourself hunting the back corners of your pantry for a cookie around 10:00 p.m., it's probably not your belly that's sending you there: It's your brain. Like a three-year-old that won't get off the swing set, your brain wants a rush—a sugar rush, that is—and it will put up a fuss until it gets it.

In fact, it's insulin—the hormone responsible for sweeping sugar out of the blood (and, often, storing it as fat)—that your brain wants to generate, according to recent studies. Sugary foods spike insulin; researchers at New York University reported that when insulin spikes, it triggers the release of dopamine, the neurotransmitter that controls the brain's reward and pleasure centers. The more insulin that's in play, the more dopamine that's released, according to 2015 animal studies reported in the journal *Nature Communications.*

But there are ways to raise dopamine levels and prevent those sugar cravings. In particular, the amino acid tyrosine (a building block of protein) has been shown to encourage the brain to release dopamine and another neurotransmitter, norepinephrine. The best sources of tyrosine:

Eggs

Spirulina
(a high-protein seaweed supplement)

Cheese
(particularly Parmesan, Gruyère, Swiss, and Romano cheese)

Milk

Sesame seeds

Beef

Bacon

ful have, on average, an extra pound of fat inside their bellies than those who are more in tune with their everyday lives and the world around them.

And *Zero Sugar Diet* teaches us to be particularly mindful of what's going into our mouths. By causing a shift from sugary, processed foods to more natural, fiber-rich whole foods, we're not just cutting sugar and boosting fiber; we're reducing our intake of other chemicals that aren't actually food, but that we eat almost every day.

In fact, "ultra-processed" foods now make up more than half of all calories consumed in the United States, according to a 2016 report in the online journal *BMJ Open*. And that, by the way, is where 90 percent of all our added sugar comes from. "Ultra-processed" means any product that uses a non-food substance (preservatives, emulsifiers, artificial flavorings) that you simply wouldn't use in a recipe you were making from scratch.

Thanks in great part to our overreliance on these products, a 2016 study in *Mayo Clinic Proceedings* found that less than 3 percent of Americans live what the authors dubbed a "healthy lifestyle." (Yes,

---

ZERO SUGAR SUCCESS STORY

Lisa Gardner, forty-nine, Elgin, SC:

"I lost ten pounds! And the diet is easy!"

Starting weight: **135** | Four weeks later: **126**

I'm a teacher in South Carolina and lost ten pounds—plus, I'm enjoying more energy and a flatter tummy. I find it easy to check labels and continue the rule, checking for sugar and fiber. The best part is, I don't need sugar, or crave desserts. Thank you so much. I will continue to follow the Zero Sugar way of life!

that number is correct: less than 3 percent.) Primarily, that's because of our processed food intake and our overall body fat. Although the vast majority of us have long ago given up smoking, and nearly half of us exercise at least two and a half hours a week, we still eat poorly, and we're still too heavy. As a result, the average American's risk of metabolic syndrome—a combination of insulin insensitivity, high cholesterol, high blood pressure, and too much abdominal fat—is unique among the global citizenry. In a 2013 study from the Institute of Health, Americans ranked dead last—literally—among seventeen First-World countries studied, at just about every stage of life, from infancy to old age, suffering from heart disease, lung disease, obesity, and diabetes at rates far above those experienced by other countries.

No Crashes,
No Cravings!

So it's not the spoonful of honey you drip into your cereal or the cube of sugar you melt in your tea that's doing most of the damage; it's all the sugar you eat that you don't even know about, sugar snuck into fruit snacks and meat dishes and tomato products. One in every 5 calories in ultra-processed foods comes from added sugar. That's why simply reading labels helped the test panel have such a dramatic impact on their weight—and their sugar cravings. "As a sugar junkie, I am amazed that it has been relatively easy to change my eating plan and reduce my sugar consumption drastically," says Elaine Grohol, fifty-eight, of Orlando, Florida, who lost 10 pounds.

Without that constant influx of added sugar coming at us in our breakfast bread, our lunch meats, and our pasta sauce at dinner, cravings become much easier to manage. "I am finding I don't crave sweets like I used to," says Kay Fritsch, fifty-eight, of Dodgeville, Wisconsin. And it doesn't hurt to have a delicious, no-sugar-added substitute: "I got the plant protein powder and those smoothies seem to help with wanting desserts," she adds.

Indeed, besides your shrinking belly, a reduction in cravings may be the single best indicator that *Zero Sugar Diet* is changing your body in significant ways. Consider this: New research from Australia shows that just three junk-food binges a week—even if you eat healthfully every other day—are enough to damage your overall gut health.

While the study was conducted on rats, research has repeatedly

5 BIZARRE WAYS TO CUT SUGAR CRAVINGS

Throw Up Your Hands

Australian researchers say that the more decisions you have to make at work each day, the more likely you are to have a larger waistline.

The study, published in *Social Science and Medicine*, found that those who have high levels of what's called "skill discretion"—i.e., they exercise control by getting things done themselves—tended to have lower BMIs. But those who are constantly deciding on courses of action for others may eventually come down with what's known as

"decision fatigue." Your sharply reasoned thought processes get worn down until you finally hit dinner time and think, *Screw it, let's just have dessert*.

Tamp Down Your Dreams

It's okay to dream big, but when it comes to weight loss, you might be better off dreaming about yourself growing big.

A study in the journal *Cognitive Therapy and Research* found that obese women who fantasized about losing weight and showing off

their hot new bodies lost an average of twenty-four fewer pounds than those who harbored negative thoughts—like how terrible they might look if they kept eating poorly. The researchers speculated that negative fantasies about weight loss prepared the dieters to overcome the bumps they encountered on their road to getting healthy.

Instagram Your Meals

We all have annoying relatives who can't eat a Big Mac without posting a picture of it first. But those who hunger for social media foodie fame might be on to something.

shown that the human gut—a giant convention center packed with a hundred trillion microbial cells—behaves much the same way. In a study, researchers compared the bellies of obese rats with those that were fed a healthy diet but were allowed to binge on sweets for a weekend. After they satisfied their cravings, the binge-diet rats had

An analysis of "attentive eating" studies in *The American Journal of Clinical Nutrition* found that those who recall their last meal as being filling and satisfying tended to eat less at their next meal. So if you're one of those people who can't remember what they had for dinner last night, start building a photo journal of your munchies, and you may soon be snapping more than just photos—like maybe a new pair of skinny jeans.

Hang Up a Mirror— in the Kitchen

Sure, you look sexy in an apron. But that's not why you should reflect on yourself when you're cooking.

In a 2015 study in the *Journal of the Association for Consumer Research*, scientists had subjects choose either a fruit salad or a chocolate cake, then eat and evaluate their snack. Those who ate the chocolate cake in the room with the mirror found it less appealing than those who didn't have a looking glass nearby. But those who chose the fruit salad reported no difference in taste; in other words, the presence of a mirror makes unhealthy foods less appealing.

Fantasize About Overeating

This might sound counterintuitive, but if you can envision yourself gorging on a sugary treat,

you might wind up eating less of it.

In one study, researchers broke participants into two groups. One group was asked to fantasize about eating three M&M'S. The other group was told to imagine themselves eating thirty. Then, the scientists invited the subjects to enjoy some real M&M'S as part of a "taste test." Strangely enough, those who fantasized about eating thirty candies actually tended to eat less of the real thing than those who kept their imaginations limited to just three. Contrary to popular belief, imagining the pleasure of gorging on a food actually reduces your appetite for it, the researchers said.

belly biomes almost identical to those of the perpetually unhealthy, obese rats.

Why is cutting cravings so critical? Because healthy microbes are responsible in part for metabolizing flavonoids, the six thousand different nutrients found in fruits and vegetables that do everything from bolstering the immune system to revving the metabolism. Once you damage the microbes lining the gut by binging on sugary foods, you damage the body's ability to absorb flavonoids—leading to a potential long-term impact on your health and your body weight. Indeed, in a study of nearly thirty-five thousand women, those with the highest intake of flavonoids over sixteen years had the lowest incidence of heart disease. (Apples, pears, red wine, grapefruit, and strawberries were among the most potent flavonoid vehicles.) A 2014 study in *The Journal of Nutrition* found that high levels of flavonoids seem to help regulate blood glucose levels, while another study found that they can reduce our incidence and severity of inflammatory diseases such as allergies, asthma, psoriasis, and, yes, obesity.

And no sugar cravings means no sugar crashes, either. Indeed, one of the main reasons panelists cited for wanting to take part in the test panel was "to feel better/have more energy." And in that, *Zero Sugar Diet* delivered. "Yes, I have more energy, I'm sleeping better, and I'm getting compliments on how 'beautiful' my skin is!" says Lynn Driscoll, fifty-eight, of Boston, Massachusetts. "Overall I feel much better physically and mentally."

"I feel better, eat less, and I have no desire to eat sweets," says teacher Lisa Gardner, forty-nine, of Elgin, South Carolina.

Wendy Hardcastle of Columbus, Georgia, reports that she's "not hungry all the time anymore," while fellow Georgian Tracey Lee says, "I don't feel as tired as I have in the past." These folks have taken back control of their bodies, their waistlines, and their energy levels by stripping out the addictive added sugars food manufacturers have been sneaking into our diets. As a result, they're no longer slaves to uncontrollable hunger, sugar crashes, and the inevitable weight gain that results. And once you can eliminate those elements from your life, once you put yourself, and not the food manufacturers, back in charge of your life, that body you've always wanted can finally become yours.

"I have not been as hungry especially in the evening, which is when I usually want to snack," says Brenda Huey of Bernville, Pennsylvania. "The flat belly is real and attainable."

Yes it is. And in the coming chapter, I'm going to show you how to make that dream a reality for yourself, as well.

chapter **6**

MAKE ZERO SUGAR DIET WORK FOR YOU

ZERO SUGAR DIET is actually composed of two phases: Phase one is a fourteen-day plan, a simple dietary reset that will detox your body, bring your hormones into balance, heal your liver, and take away your food cravings while delivering rapid weight loss. Phase two is what I call the Zero Sacrifice for Life program, designed to ease you back into your regular way of eating while you continue to lose weight. More important, it's designed to continue protecting you from the damaging effects of sugar, so that you can enjoy all your favorite foods without having to watch your calorie intake and without having to worry about gaining back weight and putting your health at risk.

Why two phases? It's simple.

First, science tells us that by reducing sugar in our diet, we can quickly and dramatically alter our physical, mental, and emotional health. There is simply so much evidence piling up that we can change the course of our health in just two weeks or less that it makes no sense to drag our feet. Do you want to henpeck the dragon to death, or slay it with one mighty blow?

But more important, I want to give you rapid belly-flattening results that will keep you motivated, because despite the common perception that you need to drop pounds slowly in order to maintain your weight loss, the exact opposite is true. In fact, you're more than five times as likely to succeed in your long-term weight-loss goals if you start out of the gate by dropping pounds rapidly, according to a 2013 study in the *International Journal of Behavioral Medicine.*

The same results have been repeated over and over again. A 2014 study in *The Lancet* looked at two hundred people on weight-loss plans and found that "achieving a weight loss target of 12.5 percent [of body weight] is more likely, and drop-out is lower, if losing weight is done quickly." And a similar study in the *Journal of Nutrition Education and Behavior* found that subjects who were more successful in the initial weeks of a weight-loss program were far more likely to stay motivated, and go on to lose at least 5 percent of their body weight, than those who started more slowly. Sorry, Mr. Tortoise, but in the weight loss Olympics, slow and steady does not win the race.

Plus, taking two weeks to focus on a small number of core foods will train you to build a simpler diet. A 2015 study at the Friedman School of Nutrition Science and Policy at Tufts University found that while most doctors subscribe to the notion of "all things in moderation," that long-standing bit of advice is actually wrong. When researchers looked at the diets of 6,814 people, they found that the more diverse one's diet, the more likely one was to experience weight gain. In fact, those who ate the widest range of foods showed a 120 percent greater increase in waist circumference compared with those who had the least diversity. In other words, people who have the best success at weight loss pick a set number of foods and tend to stick to them.

At the same time, as the saying goes, Ya gotta live. And more important, ya gotta live in twenty-first-century America, which means that your diet will—no, must—include things that don't belong in those first fourteen days. There will be days when the kids must have their Burger King, and you do, too. There will be nights when one more beer and two more handfuls of chips are gonna happen, no matter what. Children will keep having birthdays, offices will keep having Christmas parties, bars will keep having margarita happy hours, and Ben and Jerry will keep coming out with new flavors that you have to try. And NONE of those foods, I assure you, will fall into the Sweet Spot.

That's where phase two comes in: The Zero Sacrifice for Life. Using the guidelines of this maintenance program, you'll still get to enjoy the birthday cake, the margaritas, those bacon-wrapped date thingies, and the latest offerings from your ice-cream shop. Because the reality of life is this: The world is full of sugar, and it's nearly impossible to prevent yourself from eating too much of it. But what is possible is to prevent your body from suffering the full impact of it. The Zero Sacrifice for Life plan is like a sugar-immunization program that allows you to venture into danger zones safely, while others must walk in fear. Here's an overview of both phases.

The Fourteen-Day Zero Sugar

The first fourteen days on this plan are as close to a traditional "diet" as you'll ever need to come.

You will find it remarkably effective and surprisingly easy. So much so, in fact, that you may want to stay on it for even longer than fourteen days. Or, because of its insanely rapid results, you may want to return to it from time to time, in advance of a big wedding or a beach vacation.

And that's fine. When I began *Zero Sugar Diet*, and saw for myself how quickly and effectively it stripped off the pounds, I realized that eating according to this plan was changing my body in ways I never imagined possible. And I found that once I got used to reading labels a bit more carefully, I learned how much I had been sabotaging my own weight-loss goals with foods that were low in calories but that were bombarding me with added sugars. You'll find that, too. During these fourteen days, you'll discover new products and new brands that will become staples of your diet and that of your family.

Because on the first fourteen days, you'll eat only foods that have *no* added sugars. You'll enjoy eating four times a day: breakfast, lunch, dinner, and one Zero Sugar snack. There's no counting calories or worrying about whether you're eating too much or too little. The foods you'll eat on *Zero Sugar Diet* will keep you naturally satiated by stabilizing your blood sugar, filling your belly, and keeping your hunger hormones under control.

Here are the ground rules:

1. Eat foods with no added sugars, choosing from the list in the back of the book or checking nutrition labels.

2. In the coming chapters, you'll find twenty-eight homemade (but easy to make) and "semi-homemade" (using some of the best packaged foods out there) meals and snacks that will satisfy you. If you like variety, try something new every day of the week. Creature of habit? Nothing wrong with eating the same meals fourteen days in a row.

3. Phase 1 of *Zero Sugar Diet* is focused on helping you increase fiber, decrease blood sugar, and end cravings by always keeping you in the Sweet Spot, so you never eat more sugar than fiber. Stick with it to get the biggest benefit—you will have the opportunity to mix things up a bit in phase two.

4. I've tailored each meal and snack so that the carbs always have less sugar than fiber for optimal satisfaction and balance. For these fourteen days, I recommend using the suggested portion sizes in order to cut your dependence on carbs.

5. Power Proteins—foods like grilled chicken, broiled salmon, sautéed shrimp, and cubed tofu (protein foods that have nothing added, except perhaps a minimal amount of fat for cooking)—are free. So, too, are vegetables, fruits, and Flat-Belly Fats like olive, canola, avocado, and walnut oils, plant-fat rich foods like avocados and olives, and nut and seed butters like peanut butter, almond butter, and tahini. (But as with any packaged food, make sure you're looking for one with less sugar than fiber.)

6. If the prescribed serving sizes aren't cutting it for you, increase your portions of whole vegetables, fruits, and pure protein. The fiber in produce and protein are both major factors in satiety, and getting enough at each meal will help you rein in your hunger.

SAMPLE BREAKFASTS

The Zero Sugar Chocolate Smoothie

½ banana

+ ¼ ripe avocado, peeled, pitted, and quartered

+ ½ cup unsweetened coconut milk

+ ¼ cup unsweetened plant-based protein powder
  (with no artificial sweetener)

+ 6 ice cubes

+ 2 Tbsp unsweetened cocoa powder

+ Water to blend (optional)

300 calories | 11 g fat (3 g saturated) | 11 g fiber | 9 g natural sugar
25 g protein

Peanut Butter O!

½ cup rolled oats, prepared with water

+ 2 Tbsp Smucker's natural peanut butter

+ ½ cup raspberries

397 calories | 19.1 g fat (2.5 g saturated) | 108 mg sodium | 41 g carbs
10.1 g fiber | 4.1 g natural sugar | 13.1 g protein

The Good Egg

2 large eggs omelet with 2 cups baby spinach

+ 2 slices Ezekiel 4:9 sprouted whole-grain bread

+ 2 Tbsp mashed avocado

+ sea salt

354 calories | 14.5 g fat (3.9 g saturated) | 807 mg sodium | 34.5 g carbs
8.5 g fiber | 1.1 g natural sugar | 14.7 g protein

Protein Pancakes

1 medium banana, mashed

+ 2 eggs, whisked

+ 2 Tbsp ground flaxseed

+ ⅓ cup Bob's Red Mill oat bran cereal, cooked in 1 Tbsp coconut oil (serves two)

286 calories | 14.6 g fat (7.9 g saturated) | 64 mg sodium | 29.3 g carbs
6.9 g fiber | 7.7 g natural sugar | 11 g protein

Instant Breakfast

1 cup Post Shredded Wheat

+ ½ cup blackberries

+ ½ cup unsweetened almond milk

+ 2 Tbsp hemp seeds

305 calories | 10 g fat (0.4 g saturated) | 91 mg sodium | 48.9 g carbs
10.8 g fiber | 3.5 g natural sugar | 12.5 g protein

On-the-Go Options (for Phase Two only)

McDonald's
Sausage Biscuit with Egg

Dunkin' Donuts
Turkey Sausage Flatbread Sandwich

Burger King
BK Breakfast Muffin Sandwich Sausage and Cheese

LUNCH

Big Salmon Salad

4 cups romaine lettuce

+ ½ medium cucumber, chopped

+ ½ cup cherry tomatoes

+ ½ cup cooked wheat berries

+ 4 oz Bumble Bee salmon pouch

+ 2 tsp chopped parsley

+ 1 Tbsp extra-virgin olive oil

+ lemon juice

399 calories | 17.2 g fat (2.2 g saturated) | 380 mg sodium | 35.7 g carbs
3.4 g fiber | 5.9 g natural sugar | 34.5 g protein

Hummus Picnic

Single serving Sabra hummus

+ 2 Triscuits

+ ½ orange bell pepper, sliced

+ 2 stalks celery, sliced

+ 1 single serving olives

+ 100 calorie pack Emerald Nuts

265 calories | 18.5 g fat (2.2 g saturated) | 410 mg sodium | 19.6 g carbs
7.8 g fiber | 4 g natural sugar | 6.8 g protein

Roast Beef Wrap

1 Ezekiel 4:9 whole-grain tortilla

+ 2 oz deli roast beef

+ 2 tsp horseradish sauce

+ 2 romaine lettuce leaves

+ side of 1 cup grape tomatoes

349 calories | 13.4 g fat (5.9 g saturated) | 207 mg sodium | 33.3 g carbs
7.2 g fiber | 4.8 g natural sugar | 24.8 g protein

Instant Lunch

2 cups Amy's lentil soup

+ green salad with extra-virgin olive oil and lemon juice

460 calories | 17 g fat (3.2 g saturated) | 1,215 mg sodium | 57.8 g carbs
13.1 g fiber | 6.8 g natural sugar | 18.2 g protein

On-the-Go Options (for Phase Two only)

Burger King

Chicken Caesar garden fresh salad wrap, grilled

Starbucks

Zesty chicken and black bean salad bowl

Wendy's

Large chili

DINNER

Spice-Rubbed Chicken

1 Tbsp garlic powder

+ 1 Tbsp paprika, sprinkled on both sides of
1 4-oz chicken breast, grilled

+ 4 cups cauliflower florets roasted with
1 Tbsp sunflower oil

423 calories | 24.5 g fat (3 g saturated) | 179 mg sodium
8.5 g fiber | 8 g natural sugars | 34 g protein

Beefy Broccoli

3 oz skirt steak cut into thin slices stir-fried in
1 tsp sesame oil

+ 3 cups broccoli florets

+ 1 Tbsp soy sauce

+ ½ cup brown rice

425 calories | 14.9 g fat (4.8 g saturated) | 755 mg sodium | 42.1 g carbs
8.9 g fiber | 5.3 g natural sugars | 33.7 g protein

Mushroom Farrotto

1 cup cooked farro

+ 4 cups button mushrooms, sautéed with garlic and
1 tsp extra-virgin olive oil

+ ¼ cup canned white cannellini beans

+ 1 cup baby arugula

404 calories | 8 g fat (1 g saturated) | 247 mg sodium
14 g fiber | 8 g natural sugar | 24 g protein

Instant Dinner

Whole Foods frozen ahi tuna burger

+ Ezekiel 4:9 sprouted whole-grain English muffin

+ 1 romaine lettuce leaf

+ 1 tomato slice

+ 1 red onion slice

+ 1 tsp olive oil–based mayo

+ green salad

+ 1 tsp extra-virgin olive oil

+ lemon juice

351 calories | 12.5 g fat (2.3 g saturated) | 315 mg sodium | 33.2 g carbs
2.6 g fiber | 3.4 g natural sugar | 28.3 g protein

On-the-Go Options (for Phase Two only)

Applebee's

Shrimp and broccoli cavatappi

Chili's

Fresh Tex lighter choices 6-ounce sirloin with grilled avocado

Olive Garden

Grilled chicken Caesar salad

SNACKS (add in whole fruits and vegetables as needed)

SPICY:

½ cup Nature's Path Smart Bran cereal

+ 2 Tbsp peanuts

+ a pinch of chili powder

200 calories | 9.6 g fat (1.4 g saturated) | 122 mg sodium | 26.1 g carbs
5.7 g fiber | 11.2 g natural sugar | 7.2 g protein

SWEET:

½ cup Nature's Path Smart Bran cereal

+ 32 60% cacao dark chocolate chips

175 calories | 6.1 g fat (3.5 g saturated) | 117 mg sodium | 31 g carbs
6 g fiber | 16.5 g natural sugar | 3.5 g protein

INSTANT SNACKS

Chia Warrior bar, coconut flavor
The Good Bean, sea salt, 1 ounce

THE ZERO SACRIFICE FOR LIFE PLAN

Now that you've cut your dependence on added and refined sugars by eliminating them entirely, it's time to step back and let your instincts run the show. Wait, you're thinking—my instincts used to drive me straight to the vending machine at 3:00 p.m. and to Krispy Kreme every time I was at the airport. And that may be true. But you've worked hard to reset your eating tendencies. Now is the time to see how much you've learned and reap the benefits. This phase gives you total autonomy over what you eat, a crucial factor in sustained weight loss. A 2012 study in the *International Journal of Behavioral Nutrition and Physical Activity* found that if you feel autonomous—in other words, like you have total control and don't need to rely on me or my book— you are more likely to see long-lasting health changes.

For this phase of *Zero Sugar Diet*, we're focused on sustainability—

RESTAURANT RULES

Diets don't work in the long run unless they're sustainable, which is why we encourage you to take this Zero Sugar show on the road. But we also don't want out-of-the-house meals to derail your progress. Here are a few basic pointers that will help you dine in slimming style:

- If nutrition information is available, try to stick with meals that are no more than 500–600 calories. Read the menu online ahead of time so you know what you're ordering.

- If the restaurant simply doesn't offer enough choices that stack up fiber-wise, or if it hides its sugar content or other nutritional information—Cheesecake Factory, Long John Silver's, and Starbucks are among the chains that either hide their nutritionals altogether or offer a partial list that doesn't include sugar content—play it safe by noshing on a Zero Sugar Cheat Pack before heading out to the restaurant.

- No nutrition stats to be found? No problem. Start with a vegetable-based soup or salad to curb your appetite and fill half your plate with produce.

- Stick with pure proteins: meat, fish, and more that have been prepared without the addition of breading, sauces, and oils.

making health-promoting, weight-loss-inducing eating work for you over the long term. With that goal in mind, there is only one word you need to remember: fiber.

Aiming to eat 30 grams of fiber per day (or 40 if you're a man) can help you slim down, decrease blood pressure, and improve your body's response to insulin—just as effectively as following a more complicated diet, according to a study from the University of Massachusetts Medical School. The study, published in the *Annals of Internal Medicine*, tracked 240 overweight volunteers with metabolic syndrome (high blood pressure, blood sugar, and cholesterol).

ZERO SUGAR CHEAT PACKS

Throughout the Zero Sugar test panel, I communicated with our testers on nearly a daily basis, listening to their recommendations for how to make the program even easier and more foolproof. And one of the questions I got asked the most was this: "I'm going to a luncheon/dinner party/work event and I don't know what's going to be in the food. How can I make sure I'm staying in my Sweet Spot?"

Whether you're cooking at home, eating a prepackaged meal, or dining at a popular restaurant, getting a full handle on the sugar-fiber ratio is pretty easy. But once you step into uncharted territory, from catered events to your aunt Bea's home cooking, you can never be sure exactly how much sugar is being added into the sauce. So to ensure you stay in the Sweet Spot, even when you're not sure what's coming, I created a series of Zero Sugar Cheat Packs. Buy, or simply whip up, one of these versatile, on-the-go snacks, and "pregame" your meals whenever you're not sure what you'll be eating. Since each delivers a solid dose of fiber and zero sugar, eating one of these at least twenty minutes before your next mystery meal will ensure that even a too-sweet snack won't damage your liver or cause fat storage.
(**Note:** It takes twenty minutes for your body to register that

When researchers assigned people to be on either the high-fiber regimen or an American Heart Disease diet—a plan that required participants to eat more vegetables, fruits, fiber, fish, and lean protein, and less salt, sugar, fat, and alcohol—subjects in both groups had similar results, from weight loss to decreases in metabolic syndrome markers. They were also all able to maintain weight loss for twelve months.

No doubt, it's easier to follow a plan that says "Eat More X" than it is to follow one with a laundry list of rules. If the results are the same, sticking with the simpler plan is a no brainer. What's more, research

you've consumed food, which means you'll enter the dietary danger zones not only filled with healthy fiber, but less hungry than you'd otherwise be.)

And since they're portable, you can stash them in your desk or your car or your briefcase, and snack away whenever you're faced with a dicey dietary dilemma. Think of them as invisible force fields that protect your body from the damaging effects of sugar.

Plus, as you read more about the Zero Sacrifice for Life plan— the simple eating guidelines that keep the pounds melting away long after the dramatic changes of the first fourteen days—you'll see how these low-calorie, fiber-filled Cheat Packs can be used to make every day a perfect day of eating. Any time you're faced with a confusing menu—or falling victim to the siren song of sugar—eating a Cheat Pack first will not only contain your appetite but also keep your fiber intake in the healthy range.

Ak Mak sesame wheat crackers, 1 oz (5 crackers): 5 g fiber
Gemini tigernuts, ½ oz: 5 g fiber
Carrington Farms flax packs: 3 g fiber
The Chia Company chia shots: 6 g fiber
Nature's Path Smartbran, ¼ cup: 6.5 g fiber
Nature's Path Qi'a Superfood, 2 Tbsp: 4 g fiber
Kellogg's All Bran Buds, 2 Tbsp: 5 g fiber
Kellogg's All Bran original, ¼ cup: 5 g fiber
The Good Bean, sea salt, 1 oz: 5 g fiber

from Cornell University tells us that, for most people, it's more effective to focus on the positive "shoulds" of eating well rather than the "should nots."

The reason why "more fiber" works is more than just psychology, however. Indeed, just two days of eating a diet high in fiber can alter your gut biome enough to reduce inflammation and begin bodily changes that lead to weight loss, according to a 2015 study in the *American Journal of Physiology*. In fact, the authors found that adding "soluble fibers to processed foods, including calorically rich obesogenic foods, may be a means to ameliorate their detrimental effects." Just eating more fiber helps so much, you barely need to worry about what else you're eating.

And what makes this plan so easy to stick to is that high-fiber foods are uber filling. When used smartly (see below), high-fiber foods satisfy you, crowding out more caloric, less nutritious choices along the way.

Done with the first fourteen days? Now detoxed from sugar, you can continue to lose weight, and live your happiest and healthiest life. Simply follow the Zero Sugar plan but allow yourself:

CHEAT PACKS

Our sweet, salty low-sugar, high-fiber mixes will fill you up fast.

CHEAT MEALS

Eat whatever you want for two meals a week—yes, even ice cream!

ALCOHOL

Enjoy—but no more than one glass a day, max. We'd recommend no more than that even if you weren't following this diet.

But don't be surprised if you find yourself not wanting too many sweets. After two weeks on *Zero Sugar Diet*, test panelists reported a decreased desire for sugary foods. That's just one of the long-lasting benefits of finding your Sweet Spot.

chapter

7

A DAY OF EATING THE ZERO SUGAR WAY

WHEN WAS THE LAST TIME YOU ATE OUT? Chances are you said last night. Like most Americans, you might get about 43 percent of your calories from outside the home, or about 799 calories of restaurant- or store-prepared foods each day. (In the 1980s, the average American got just 20 percent of his or her calories from outside the home, according to the USDA.) And access to restaurant foods has only gotten easier, thanks to GrubHub and Seamless, Yelp and Open-

Table, the growing food truck industry, and the larger and larger sections of grocery stores and even Costco that are dedicated to rotisserie chickens and other premade fare.

That's part of why we've grown heavier: In a 2014 study in the journal *Public Health Nutrition,* people were asked to report their food intake over the course of forty-eight hours. Those who ate at a restaurant during that time took in an average of 200 calories per day more than those who prepared all their own meals. (Those who ate in sit-down restaurants actually consumed slightly more calories than those who ordered from fast-food joints.)

And if you are an average American woman, you, too, struggle with your weight. Let's say you weigh 166 pounds. (That, by the way, is about 10 pounds heavier than the average American woman in 1996, and just about what the average American man weighed in the early 1960s.) Perhaps your waist is 37.5 inches—again, average for an American woman circa 2016, according to the Centers for Disease Control and Prevention. (The average American man is 195.5 pounds and has a waist circumference of 39.7 inches.)

In other words, like 69 percent of Americans over the age of twenty, there's a chance you're overweight. So you've probably done what people do when they start to worry about their weight: Try to watch what you eat.

But watching what you eat is one thing; knowing exactly what to watch for when you eat is the real challenge. We've been told so many things over the years, from "eat less fat" to "eat low carb"—and that's just from the U.S. government. And we've been (literally) fed dozens of diet fads, from juice cleanses to gluten-free plans to Paleo programs. It's no wonder that a survey by the International Food Information Council Foundation found that three out of four people felt like all the changes in nutrition advice made it hard to know what to eat, and 52 percent said it was easier to do their own taxes than it was to pick healthy foods.

The Amazing Secret
to Eating Well

What makes us gain weight?

If you said "calories," you're right. But also, you're not right.

If cutting calories were all it took to lose weight—simply exercising a little more, or eating a little less—then weight loss would be as simple as third-grade math: Subtract y from z and end up with x.

But if you've followed any diet or exercise program and achieved less than the desired result, you've probably come away frustrated, depressed, maybe feeling a little guilty—and angry, too. Instead of permanent weight loss, we get temporary results and long-term failure. Instead of x, we get xxl. Why?

Because there's more at work than just calories in and calories out. And while it's easier than ever to know how many calories are in your order, that also means that it's easier than ever to fall into the trap of counting only calories, and not focusing on sugar and fiber. Writing in the journal *Open Heart* in 2015, scientists estimated that replacing low-calorie foods with two servings of fatty, high-calorie (and high-fiber) nuts a week could save ninety thousand lives in the United States every year.

Our bodies are like magnificent, and mysterious, ecosystems. They evolved to have a certain balance of nutrients, and that balance helps to determine the functions of our hormones and our gut biomes. When that balance is thrown off, a lot of crazy starts to happen. And that often leads to weight gain and health risks.

For example, one of the most powerful contributors to weight loss is a compound called butyrate, a fatty acid that's produced in your colon by a your gut bacteria, in particular the family Bacteriodetes, feasting on fiber. Butyrate promotes weight loss and reduces inflammation by deactivating the genes linked to obesity and inflammatory response—and in doing so, it also reduces our risk of heart disease, diabetes, arthritis, and many other inflammation-related diseases.

But a recent study found that when people lose weight through a low-calorie diet, the results included an increase in the bacterial family Firmacutes—the enemies of our healthy gut bacteria—and a reduction in the body's levels of butyrate. That's part of the reason why energy-restrictive diets lead to long-term weight gain: They kill off our healthy gut bacteria.

And in another study in Australia, researchers looked at different kinds of diets, including low-sugar and high-protein diets, to see if they made a difference in how the dieters' bodies reacted. They put all of the subjects on the same number of calories, and broke them into four groups, trying out variations on high- and low-protein and high- and low-sugar plans. They found that all things being equal, reducing sugar helped people lose weight faster, even when overall calories remained the same. "[R]apidly digestible [carbs] can cause marked fluctuations in blood glucose and insulin levels, in turn stimulating hunger and inhibiting fat oxidation [i.e., fat burning]." They concluded that while high-protein and low-sugar diets both increased body fat loss, a high-carb, low-sugar diet was the best for cutting both fat and cardiovascular risk.

In other words, trying to reduce calories in order to lose weight doesn't work, because there are too many other factors at play. It's like trying to row a boat with one oar. Worse, in fact, because not only does calorie reduction send you around and around in a lose-gain circle, but in the long run it causes you to gain more weight than you lost.

A DAY OF PERFECT EATING

Let's think about two more average American women, Mary and Jane. As we said, they're both trying to watch what they eat. Here's what they ate today:

BREAKFAST:

Mary and Jane both stopped by Dunkin' Donuts on the way to work. Along with a black coffee, they also ordered breakfast.

Mary's order:
Ham, Egg, and Cheese on
an English Muffin

Jane's order:
Original Oatmeal with
Dried Fruit Topping

LUNCH:

Since they're trying to slim down, Mary and Jane are both eating healthy, low-calorie soups they brought from home. Each of the soups is under 200 calories per cup, so even though they're having two cups, they know they're not overdoing it on the calories. And they each had some fresh fruit for a healthy post-lunch dessert.

Mary:
2 cups Amy's Lentil Soup,
plus ½ cup of raspberries

Jane:
2 cups Campbell's Organic
Sun-Ripened Tomato &
Basil Bisque,
plus ½ cup of raspberries

SNACK:

These ladies are smart enough not to hit the vending machines. In fact, there's a health food store near their office. Both made the conscientious decision to pop in and buy a nutrition bar.

Mary:
Chia Warrior Bar,
coconut flavor

Jane:
KIND Bar, Fruit & Nut
Delight flavor

DINNER:

Since Mary and Jane are old friends, they decided to meet up at Applebee's for an early dinner. And since both are surreptitiously on a diet, they both ordered off the "Lite" menu.

Mary:
Applebee's
Shrimp & Broccoli
Cavatappi

Jane:
Applebee's
Cedar Grilled Lemon
Chicken

Now, here's the question: Which one of these women is actually going to lose weight?

It may seem like Mary and Jane are eating almost identical diets, and that they're both setting themselves up to look and feel leaner and healthier. In fact, Mary ate a total of 1,302 calories, while Jane ate almost the same number: 1,372. But in fact, only one of them is actually eating in a way that stabilizes her blood sugar, heals her digestive system, and allows her body to shed belly fat. And here's why calories are a terrible measure of dietary health:

Mary: 33 g fiber, 17.5 g sugar
Jane: 21 g fiber, 72.5 g sugar

Not only did Jane eat nearly four times more sugar than fiber, but the majority of the sugar she ate was added sugar: nearly three times as much as the American Heart Association, the World Health Organization, and the USDA recommend for women. And as I said earlier in the book, every 23 grams of added sugar you eat per day increases your risk of diabetes by 18 percent. That means that Jane is at a 54 percent greater risk than Mary, even though the calories they ate were nearly identical.

You see, one of the things about sugar is that it's so deceptive. It appears in surprising quantities in healthy-sounding foods, foods that most people—even nutritionally aware people—would choose as a clearly healthy option.

Jane's breakfast oatmeal, for instance, contained 22 grams of sugar—nearly a day's worth—thanks to the dried fruit, which more often than not comes coated with added sugar. (And this is before the addition of any brown sugar or maple syrup, which would add another 6 or more grams.) And while her organic tomato soup lunch sure sounds healthy, it comes with a whopping 24 grams of sugar, much of which is added; just because that sugar is organic doesn't mean it's good for you.

Mary, on the other hand, stayed in the Sweet Spot all day long. In the end, her sugar-to-fiber ratio was almost exactly one to two, putting her far ahead of the minimum ratio she needs to control her hunger and fat-storage hormones, protect her liver from damage, and prevent inflammation and weight gain. Jane, on the other hand, forced her body into fat-storage mode almost from her first bite of food; her overall ratio was a deeply unhealthy 3.5-to-1.

What did Mary do right that Jane got wrong? Let's break it down.

BREAKFAST

Cook up a container of plain oatmeal and you have a breakfast that starts your day off at a 1:4 sugar-to-fiber ratio. But oatmeal is like a blank canvas that food marketers can paint with any number of crazy caloric colors, secure in the knowledge that their product will be illuminated by a well-polished health halo. That's why McDonald's, home of the all-day breakfast, can offer a Fruit & Maple Oatmeal with 32 grams of sugar. Burger King (29 grams), Jamba Juice (25 grams), IHOP (29 grams), and Denny's (27 grams) all offer to start your morning with a day's worth of sugar in their oatmeal. And on the packaged food front, Quaker Oats has products that vary from 1 gram of sugar to 14 grams (their Real Medleys Oatmeal + Summer Berry).

The Breakfast Rules for the First Fourteen Days:

- ▶ Packaged foods—cereals, breads, waffles, etc.—should have no added sugars.

- ▶ All dairy is fine as long as it's plain; flavor it yourself.

- ▶ Add all the fresh fruit you want to any dish.

- ▶ A touch of maple syrup, honey, jam, or brown sugar is okay after the first fourteen days, as long as you're eating a fiber-rich breakfast.

LUNCH

As I stated above, "organic" does not mean very much when you're trying to reduce sugar intake. Plenty of foods use organic sugar to sweeten the deal with consumers who think they're eating healthily.

The Lunch Rules for the First Fourteen Days:

▶ Choose thick, chunky soups, which tend to be higher in fiber, and sandwiches with lean, unprocessed meats. Choose whole-grain breads and pastas, and load up on the vegetables.

▶ Avoid salad dressing unless you know what's in it. Opt for plain oil and vinegar instead. And beware of dried fruit in your salad.

▶ All packaged foods must have no added sugars.

SNACK

Snacking and weight loss go hand-in-hand. Studies show that people who consciously refrain from eating between meals may end up consuming more calories overall during the day, often because their energy stores run low, and that leads them to make bad choices.

And bad choices sometimes look like good choices: While KIND bars have long been one of my go-to snacks, I've become more wary of them in recent years. While the sugars in the bars come from real fruit, they still count as a packaged food, which means you should only accept products that come with less sugar than fiber.

The Snack Rules for the First Fourteen Days:

▶ Fruit and other whole foods are the best snacks.

▶ Dairy is fine as long as there are no added sugars.

▶ All packaged foods must have no added sugars.

DINNER

Let's face it, dinner is a celebration at least half of the times we sit down to eat. We're with friends, we're with family, the game is on—something's happening that makes dinnertime different from other meals. During your first fourteen days, you'll be avoiding dessert entirely, but after that, you'll be focusing on adding fiber, fiber, fiber.

The Dinner Rules:

▶ Most of the rules that apply to lunch apply here as well.

▶ Make lean meats and vegetables at least two-thirds of your plate.

▶ Try to have beans or lentils plus whole grains twice a week, fish twice a week, poultry once or twice a week, and leave one or two days for your favorite red meat.

Special Report

THE CHASE FOR THE ZERO SUGAR VACCINE

WHAT DO TONY ORLANDO, J. Edgar Hoover, and your mom all have in common? Whether they know it or not, each has played a small role in helping to try to cure diabetes. And if recent breakthroughs are any indication, their work may soon be coming to fruition.

If a cure for diabetes is on the imminent horizon, it may be thanks in part to the Fraternal Order of Eagles (FOE), a charity organization that counts celebrities (like Orlando) and government leaders (like Hoover) among its alumni, and which, until recently, was most famous for helping to found Mother's Day back in 1914. But in 2014, the charity organization known for promoting motherhood raised $25 million to help build the FOE Diabetes Research Center on the campus of the University of Iowa, a twenty-thousand-square-foot advanced science facility staffed by one hundred researchers and an army of UI students all working toward a common goal. Orlando, the "Tie a Yellow Ribbon" singer and FOE member, was even on hand for the grand opening.

The facility is flooded with bright, natural light, and flooded as well with bright grad students who understand the urgency of their mission. Between 1980 and 2014, the number of adults in the United States with newly diagnosed diabetes more than tripled, according to the Centers for Disease Control, with about 1.4 million new cases each year. And as sugar continues to flood our food supply, the question of how to help our bodies overcome it grows more urgent.

A cage full of big, fat mice might have the answer.

The End Of Obesity?

They call it the Potthoff Lab, named after Matthew Potthoff, PhD, the young, lean, crew cut scientist who leads a team of students in a quest to solve one of the biggest health challenges of our time.

Team Potthoff studies the endocrine system, in particular the hormones that regulate metabolism. Of late, they've begun to drill down on a very particular hormone called fibroblast growth factor 21, or

FGF21. But because fibroblast growth factors are a whole family of compounds, Potthoff just calls his favorite new hormone 21 for short.

Fibroblasts are sort of like those big mixing machines you see on a construction site; they are a type of cell that generates collagen and other types of connective tissue, the mortar that holds together the bricks of your body. The term "blast" is a biology term that means "a cell that gets stuff done." As the cells of your body age and die off, various "blasts" help rebuild them. When you lift weights and generate muscle, the same thing happens.

These fibroblasts work at the direction of a series of enzymes, called fibroblast growth factors, or FGFs—sort of the juice that turns the lights on. Most FGFs behave in very controlled ways; they are produced by one cell, and then act on a nearby cell. So an FGF that's produced in the skin might help to regenerate new skin tissue after an injury. FGFs produced in the digestive system act on liver cells.

But FGF21 is the rebel of the

family. Instead of staying local, it diffuses into the bloodstream, taking on the characteristics of a hormone—meaning it works at different places throughout the body. As it runs loose, it seems to do a lot of extraordinary things. But two of those things are perhaps the most shocking:

First, 21 improves the rate at which our bodies burn calories while at rest.

And second—and this is where Potthoff's team is making noise in the science world—21 makes us not want to eat sugar.

"Twenty-one is the most potent insulin metabolizer ever discovered," Dr. Potthoff says. "It boosts energy expenditure. Mice that have high levels of 21 can eat a high-fat diet and not gain weight. But they won't eat sweets."

Putting a Dent in Diabetes

Researchers have known since 2005 that FGF21 reduces blood glucose levels by improving insulin sensitivity—essentially reversing diabetes. But it does more than that. It essentially attacks the entire range of disorders known as "metabolic syndrome," a collection of health dangers including high cholesterol, elevated blood sugar, and weight gain. FGF21 reduces cholesterol, particularly triglycerides, by slowing the liver's generation of these unhealthy blood fats. And 21 stimulates the action of what's known as "brown fat," a type of fat cell that actually burns calories, resulting in a higher resting metabolism and, inevitably, weight loss.

These effects have been measured not only in rodents and apes but in people. In 2013, researchers working for the pharmaceutical giant Eli Lilly did an initial test of a synthetic form of FGF21 in humans; forty-six obese people who had been diagnosed with diabetes an average of eleven years prior were injected with 3, 10, or 20 milligrams a day of an FGF21-mimicking drug with the evocative name of LY2405319.

After twenty-eight days, those who received 10 or 20 milligrams per day saw their LDL cholesterol drop between 20 and 30 percent, and all three groups saw an improvement in their

HDL cholesterol of 15 to 20 percent. Fasting glucose levels fell across the board, and participants lost between 1 and 2.8 percent of their overall body fat in less than a month. They also showed improvements in their levels of adiponectin, a protein created by the fatty tissues in the body that helps to regulate glucose and break down fat.

Earlier in this book, I discussed how dietary sugar, in particular fructose, causes damage to the liver. In fact, 31 percent of adults and 13 percent of kids suffer from non-alcoholic fatty liver disease (NAFLD), according to the experts at Sugar Science, an educational website founded by researchers at the University of California, San Francisco. And it's the sugar/liver connection that may provide the clue to how we harness FGF21 to bring an end to diabetes and metabolic syndrome.

"We know that this hormone is induced by a number of things," says Dr. Potthoff, "but one of them is fatty liver. Initially 21 is functioning normally, but as you start to become obese or diabetic, 21 starts to go up—induced by liver stress."

Your body begins to react to this increase in FGF21 much as it reacts to an increase in insulin when you chronically overeat: It starts to get pissed off. Your body develops a resistance to 21, just as it develops a resistance to insulin. "We know the point at which we become 21-resistant, and it correlates with fatty liver. What we don't know is whether the relationship is causative, or correlative," Potthoff says.

"But pharmacological levels of 21 can overcome resistance to 21 [just as injections of insulin are used to treat insulin resistance]. We're talking about 10,000 times as much 21 as is natural." And the result is a body with a superhot fat-burning oven.

The exact mechanism remains unclear; the drug may be working directly on the brain itself to increase resting metabolism, or it may be working primarily on the fat cells. What we do know is this: It works almost immediately, regardless of what your diet looks like.

"It starts as early as three days in rodents," Potthoff says. "If you induce obesity in a mouse by feeding it a high-fat diet, you can reverse almost all signs of diabetes and metabolic syndrome even while they still eat a high-fat diet."

The End of Sugar Cravings

Naturally slim people—the kind of folks who can eat all day and not gain an ounce—often have unusually high levels of 21. They're the folks who won the genetic lottery, thanks to a somewhat rare, inherited change to their DNA sequence. Researchers looking at the different types of macronutrients people eat have found that those with a preference for low-carb meals are far more likely to demonstrate this particularly fortuitous gene mutation. On the other hand, those who crave sweets are often lacking in 21, or else have developed a resistance to it. "Changes in the DNA sequence in humans—natural DNA mutations that are inheritable—can create a preference for carb intake," says Dr. Potthoff.

At least, that was the theory that the Potthoff team set out to investigate.

Scientists have known for decades that certain hormones control appetite. Ghrelin, which is produced in the gastrointestinal tract when our bellies are empty, is the "I'm hungry" hormone. Leptin, produced by the fat cells, is the "I'm full" hormone. (Sadly, as we grow heavier, we can also build up a resistance to leptin, which is why overweight people are more likely to overeat.)

But the idea that a certain hormone could control not just the amount of food we want to eat but the type of food was a bizarre new twist.

To test this theory, Potthoff's team created a group of mice that lacked the gene to create FGF21. The mice showed that they would gorge themselves on sweets. Then Potthoff's team administered doses of 21 to the creatures, and suddenly the mice's cravings stopped. "When we took a purified protein and injected it into the mice, they reduced their sugar intake tenfold," Dr. Potthoff says. The mice also rejected non-caloric sweeteners. But they still ate carbohydrates; it was only the sweet-tasting foods that they rejected.

The question is, Why? Does 21 make the sugar taste bad? To find out, the Potthoff team recorded the messages sent by the chorda tympani nerve—a nerve in the tongue of both rodents and humans that transmits taste signals from the tongue to the brain. "With or without the hormone, the recordings were the same," Dr. Potthoff says. "At least on the level of the tongue, sugar is sensed the same."

Potthoff believes that FGF21 affects neurons in the hypothalamus. "The hormone is changing the interpretation in the brain. It reduces the brain's interest in eating more."

That's both the promise of FGF21 and the danger. Or, as Dr. Potthoff puts it, "If something sounds too good to be true, it probably is. And one potential side effect of 21 is that it impacts the brain's reward system." Because the brain's reward centers are no longer lit up by

sugar, the addictive, drug-like effect of sweets is broken. The question is, What else gets broken?

"Potentially, patients on this drug might become depressed, or not be able to enjoy food, sex, and other aspects of life," Potthoff says.

"Cleaning Up" After Sugar

While FGF21 continues to reveal its remarkable powers, other scientists are chasing after a different type of sugar cure: one that can undo the damage caused by sweets, in theory protecting us from the very developments that lead to FGF21 resistance in the first place.

At the University of Montreal Hospital Centre, Drs. Marc Prentki and Murthy Madiraju have discovered what Prentki calls a "glucose detoxification machine": an enzyme that seems to render this otherwise toxic blood sugar totally harmless.

When glucose rises in the body, it causes the liver to form abdominal fat and to pump out triglycerides, leading to an unhealthy amount of cholesterol in the bloodstream. But the newly discovered enzyme, G3PP, essentially diverts some of the glucose and causes it to be converted into glycerol, which is quickly and harmlessly excreted from the body.

"If you can prevent the transition of glucose into triglycerides, you could potentially prevent obesity," Dr. Prentki says. "You could halt the transition from prediabetes to diabetes."

While the discovery of G3PP is so new that studies testing its effects haven't yet been conducted, the researchers believe this could be one more approach toward curing diabetes, obesity, and most of life's other major illnesses. In fact, Prentki says, once you control glucose, you control the body's entire cell-making machine—including the machine that makes cancer cells. "What makes cancer cells grow is glucose," he explains.

Sugar, it turns out, may not just be the cause of many of our troubles. It may also be a pathway to a cure.

chapter

8

ZERO SUGAR BREAKFASTS

THE DEBATE OVER WHETHER OR NOT to eat breakfast is settled. And the correct answer is: Dig in.

For the last several years, news reports and studies have raised a question over whether breakfast really was the most important meal of the day. Various news organizations, from *The New York Times* to *The American Journal of Clinical Nutrition*, have called the practice of a morning meal into question, and new weight-loss approaches like intermittent fasting have put people off their a.m. rituals. As a result, skipping breakfast entirely—or replacing it with a cup of coffee and a pat of butter, if you're following the "Bulletproof Coffee" craze—has become a real trend among weight-loss devotees.

But when you step out of the world of theoretical science and into the real world, the proof is simply hard to deny. In 2015, researchers at Cornell University's Food & Brand Lab surveyed 147 people who have maintained a healthy weight for several years without dieting or struggle, and asked them about their breakfast habits. Only 4 percent of the slim people surveyed said they didn't eat breakfast regularly. Of those who did:

51 percent ate fruits and vegetables
41 percent ate dairy
33 percent ate cold cereal
32 percent ate bread
31 percent ate eggs
29 percent ate hot cereal
26 percent drank coffee

In other words, 96% percent of slim people eat breakfast, and the vast majority of them eat a high-fiber breakfast with protein. Not surprising, is it?

In fact, a high-fiber, high-protein breakfast may be the most important investment you can make in your waistline. That's the finding of a recent study from the University of Missouri in Columbia, which found that eating breakfast triggered women's brains to release dopamine, a feel-good chemical that helps to control impulses.

The researchers put a group of overweight women between the ages of eighteen and twenty who regularly skipped breakfast through a series of diet tests. One week they ate a breakfast high in protein; one week a breakfast with moderate amounts of protein; and the third week, they skipped breakfast entirely. Blood samples showed that eating breakfast resulted in higher dopamine levels, and the questionnaires the women filled out indicated that when they ate breakfast, they had fewer food cravings later in the day.

And if you struggle with diabetes, breakfast may be even more important, according to a 2015 study from Tel Aviv University. Researchers there put twenty-two type 2 diabetics on a two-day diet. Each day, the participants ate the same number of calories and the same balance of nutrients; the only difference was that one day the subjects ate breakfast, and on the other day they didn't eat until noon. Researchers found that on the day the subjects skipped breakfast, they experienced major blood sugar spikes throughout the day, and their insulin response was inhibited.

But unless you're self-employed or living a life of leisure, breakfast needs to be simple and convenient if it's going to be a regular part of your life. Hence, I bring you:

MAXIMIZE YOUR BREAKFAST

Stay in the Sweet Spot

As with every meal, you'll ensure that each breakfast has no added sugar for the first fourteen days and at least as much fiber as sugar after that.

But Max Your Fiber If You Can

Breakfast accounts for just 21 percent of the average person's fiber intake, versus 30 percent at lunch and 40 percent at dinner. But shifting that balance could help. Take this study with a grain of salt, because it was sponsored by Kellogg's, but it does ring true: In a study of nearly eleven thousand adults, researchers found that when people eat 3 or more grams of fiber for breakfast, they tend to take in 14 percent more fiber overall during their day.

Pack in the Protein

While your sugar-to-fiber ratio is the most important consideration, eating a protein-rich breakfast has been proven time and again to help control food cravings and reduce your total caloric intake throughout the day. In fact, don't be afraid to order the three-egg omelet: In a 2013 Israeli study of people with type 2 diabetes, those who ate a large, protein-rich breakfast were better able to control their blood sugar and blood pressure—and had their diabetes medications reduced. Those who ate a small breakfast that was light on protein were more likely to have their meds increased.

Max Your Calorie Burn

Protein may do more than stabilize your blood sugar: It may actually set you up for a more active, higher-metabolism day. A 2015 study at the University of Arkansas found that young people who ate protein for breakfast not only felt less hunger later in the day but burned more calories and broke down more fat than those who ate a carbohydrate-rich breakfast.

Burn It Off Before You Eat It Up

Working out before breakfast will help you burn more calories than exercising at lunch, according to recent studies. Scientists in Belgium divided young men into two groups and asked them to follow a diet with 30 percent more calories and 50 percent more fat than they normally ate. Half of the group exercised in the afternoon while the other half exercised before breakfast.

The men who worked out at midday gained weight—after all, upping your calorie intake by 30 percent is a pretty substantial boost, no matter what your fitness routine. But incredibly, the men who followed the same increased-calorie diet but who exercised in the morning, before breakfast, experienced no weight gain at all. They also maintained healthy insulin levels and burned more fat throughout the day than the other group.

Get a Real Egg

While a breakfast sandwich is a great low-sugar, high-protein option, it's always better to eat real food. The yellow blocks of foam we often find in fast-food breakfast sandwiches aren't real eggs at all, but this creepy thing called "egg blend," which has an ingredient list that reads like a hairspray bottle and often includes propylene glycol, a solvent also found in antifreeze. Real eggs are the healthy way to go: A study in the *International Journal of Obesity* compared a bagel-only breakfast with that of two eggs. Participants who added two eggs, daily, had an easier time sticking to their diets due to their satiety value. The good news is that you can often order a real egg, just by asking! At McDonald's, ask for a "round egg" with your order; the real-egg cue for Denny's servers is "cracked on the grill." You'll have to crack the code yourself at other establishments, but it's worth a shot.

MAKE-IT-QUICK AT-HOME BREAKFASTS

PB&R Oatmeal

½ cup rolled oats, cooked in water

+ 2 Tbsp Smucker's natural peanut butter

+ ½ cup raspberries

> 373 calories | 10 g fat (3 g saturated) | 6 g natural sugar
> 11 g fiber | 14 g protein | 157 mg sodium

Protein Pancakes

1 medium banana, mashed

+ 2 eggs, whisked

+ 2 Tbsp ground flaxseed

+ ⅓ cup Bob's Red Mill oat bran cereal, cooked in 1 Tbsp coconut oil
(serves two)

> Per serving: 286 calories | 14.6 g fat (7.9 g saturated) | 7.7 g natural sugar
> 6.9 g fiber | 11 g protein | 64 mg sodium

How Green Is My Smoothie?

¼ cup silken tofu

+ 2 kale leaves, stems trimmed

+ ½ frozen banana

+ 1 cup unsweetened almond milk

+ 2 Tbsp chia seeds

> 363 calories | 14 g fat (4 g saturated) | 10 g natural sugar
> 13 g fiber | 13 g protein | 77 mg sodium

The Pinkie Tuscadero Smoothie

¼ cup silken tofu

+ ½ cup steamed cauliflower

+ ½ cup frozen strawberries

+ 2 Tbsp tahini

+ 1 cup unsweetened almond milk

+ 1 Tbsp chia seeds

Add to blender and mix until well blended.

> 477 calories | 26 g fat (5 g saturated) | 5 g natural sugar
> 9 g fiber | 16 g protein | 91 g sodium

Banana Chia Pudding (makes 4 servings)

3 cups unsweetened almond milk

+ ½ cup chia seeds

Mix and allow to sit in fridge overnight to thicken. Serve topped with ½ small banana, mashed, and ½ tsp cinnamon.

> Per serving: 240 calories | 12 g fat (1 g saturated) | 12 g natural sugar
> 13 g fiber | 8 g protein | 0 g sodium

Strawberry Almond Overnight Oats

⅓ cup rolled oats

+ 2 Tbsp chia seeds

+ 1 cup unsweetened almond milk

+ 1 tsp vanilla extract

+ ¼ cup strawberries, sliced

+ 2 Tbsp sliced almonds

Mix the oats, chia seeds, almond milk, and vanilla.

Refrigerate overnight.

Serve topped with strawberries and almonds.

341 calories | 19 g fat (2 g saturated) | 3 g natural sugar
15 g fiber | 14 g protein | 0 mg sodium

Southwest Scramble

1 Tbsp extra-virgin olive oil

+ 2 Tbsp minced onion

+ ¼ cup diced red bell pepper

+ 2 eggs

+ ¼ cup pinto beans

+ ¼ avocado, chopped

+ 2 Tbsp cilantro

Heat the oil in a frying pan and add onion and bell pepper,
stirring until softened. Add eggs, beans, avocado, and cilantro
and cook until the eggs are cooked to your preferred consistency.

480 calories | 37.5 g fat (8 g saturated) | 5 g natural sugar
8 g fiber | 18 g protein | 349 mg sodium

Neat-o Burrito Bowl

½ cup black beans

+ ¼ cup store-bought pico de gallo

+ 1 fried egg

+ ½ avocado, cubed

> 376 calories | 22 g fat (4 g saturated) | 1 g natural sugar
> 15 g fiber | 15 g protein | 177 mg sodium

Sweet Potato Hash

½ cup cubed baked sweet potato

+ ½ cup chopped kale

+ ½ cup cooked quinoa

+ 1 Tbsp ground flaxseed

+ 1 fried egg

+ 2 tsp coconut oil

> 412 calories | 21 g fat (10 g saturated) | 8 g natural sugar
> 8 g fiber | 14 g protein | 351 mg sodium

Mediterranean Scramble

½ cup tofu, cubed

+ crushed garlic

+ 4 cups spinach, sautéed in extra-virgin olive oil spray and topped
  with ½ cup grape tomatoes, quartered

+ ¼ cup fresh basil, torn

+ 2 tsp balsamic vinegar

+ 3 Tbsp hemp seeds

> 424 calories | 32 g fat (4 g saturated) | 4 g natural sugar
> 8 g fiber | 24 g protein | 115 mg sodium

Buckwheat Berry Bowl

1 cup cooked buckwheat

+ ¼ cup unsweetened almond milk

+ ¼ tsp vanilla extract

+ ¼ cup frozen wild blueberries

+ 2 Tbsp sliced almonds

+ 1 Tbsp ground flaxseed

Mix and heat in the microwave.

> 307 calories | 12 g fat (1 g saturated) | 6 g natural sugar
> 10 g fiber | 10 g protein | 58 mg sodium

Salmon Eggs

2 eggs, scrambled

+ 2 oz canned salmon, flaked

+ ¼ avocado, cubed

+ ½ cup baby arugula

+ 1 Tbsp hemp seeds

> 496 calories | 37 g fat (7 g saturated) | 3 g natural sugar
> 8 g fiber | 30 g protein | 416 mg sodium

ON-THE-GO BREAKFASTS
(after the first fourteen days)

Fast Food

Taco Bell
Side of egg + hash browns + mild border sauce

> 220 calories | 16 g fat (2 g saturated) | 0 g sugar
> 2 g fiber | 4 g protein | 390 mg sodium

McDonald's

Scrambled eggs

150 calories | 10 g fat (3.5 g saturated) | 0 g sugar
0 g fiber | 12 g protein | 70 mg sodium

Diners

IHOP

2 fried eggs + avocado

240 calories | 19 g fat (5 g saturated) | 0 g sugar
3 g fiber | 14 g protein | 160 mg sodium

Egg omelet + spinach (add as many additional vegetables as you'd like)

545 calories | 43 g fat (11g saturated) | 1 g sugar
3 g fiber | 28 g protein | 635 mg sodium

Denny's

Fit Fare Veggie Skillet

340 calories | 11 g fat (2 g saturated) | 8 g sugar
8 g fiber | 19 g protein | 1,360 mg sodium

Bob Evans

Sunrise: Two scrambled eggs with three slices of bacon

300 calories | 21 g fat (8 g saturated) | 0 g sugar
0 g fiber | 23 g protein | 1,130 mg sodium

Oatmeal

80 calories | 1.5 g fat (0 g saturated) | 0 g sugar
2 g fiber | 7 g protein | 150 mg sodium

Sandwich and Wrap Shops

Panera Bread

Steel-cut oatmeal with strawberries and pecans; no cinnamon sugar topping

300 calories | 10 g fat (0 g saturated) | 14 g sugar
9 g fiber | 6 g protein | 150 mg sodium

Qdoba

Breakfast bowl: Grilled chicken **+** potatoes **+** mango salsa **+** salsa roja

380 calories | 13 g fat (3.5 g saturated) | 6 g sugar
7 g fiber | 26 g protein | 1,230 mg sodium

Breakfast bowl: Eggs **+** potatoes **+** salsa verde **+** pico de gallo

345 calories | 15 g fat (4.5 g saturated) | 1 g sugar
7 g fiber | 17 g protein | 1,160 mg sodium

Cosí

Egg white cup: Pico De Gallo

90 calories | 0 g fat | 0 g sugar | 1 g fiber
21 g protein | 290 mg sodium

Egg white cup: Florentine

150 calories | 6 g fat (4 g saturated) | 0 g sugar
0 g fiber | 24 g protein | 400 mg sodium

Fruit salad

84 calories | 1 g fat (0 g saturated) | 0 g sugar
2 g fiber | 2 g protein | 18 mg sodium

Steel-cut oatmeal

149 calories | 3 g fat (0 g saturated) | 3 g sugar
4 g fiber | 5 g protein | 47 mg sodium

Coffee Shops

Dunkin' Donuts

Egg white veggie flatbread

280 calories | 9 g fat (4.5 g saturated) | 3 g sugar
4 g fiber | 15 g protein | 690 mg sodium

Egg and cheese on English muffin

240 calories | 7 g fat (4.4 g saturated) | 2 g sugar
7 g fiber | 12 g protein | 470 mg sodium

Egg and cheese wake-up wrap

150 calories | 8 g fat (3.5 g saturated) | 1 g sugar
1 g fiber | 7 g protein | 420 mg sodium

Egg white veggie wake-up wrap

150 calories | 7 g fat (3 g saturated) | 1 g sugar
1 g fiber | 9 g protein | 360 mg sodium

Starbucks

Classic Whole Grain Oatmeal (add nuts and blueberries)

160 calories | 2.5 g fat (0.5 g saturated) | 0 g sugar
4 g fiber | 5 g protein | 0 mg sodium

Au Bon Pain

Classic oatmeal: Add nuts, milk, ¼ cup fresh fruit

170 calories | 3 g fat (0 g saturated) | 1 g sugar
4 g fiber | 6 g protein | 5 mg sodium

Hard-boiled eggs (2) + ½ container mixed nuts

370 calories | 31 g fat (6 g saturated) | 3 g sugar
3 g fiber | 20 g protein | 260 mg sodium

HEALTH-FOOD IMPOSTERS

Whether it's a healthy-sounding product
that's swimming in sugar or an oft-trusted brand
that fails to deliver the goods, here are a few breakfast
products that look and sound good—but will
give you nothing but a sugar crash.
(Nutritionals are for 1 cup unless otherwise indicated.)

Kashi Strawberry Fields

200 calories | 0 g fat | 11 g sugar
3 g fiber | 190 mg sodium

This is one of Kashi's biggest flops. Strawberry Fields features white rice instead of the 7 Whole Grain blend found in many of its cereals.

Post Honey Bunches of Oats with Real Strawberries

160 calories | 2 g fat (0 g saturated) | 11 g sugar
3 g fiber | 167 mg sodium

This bowl-and-spoon treat is far too heavy on the carbs to be considered a smart pick.

General Mills Apple Cinnamon Cheerios

160 calories | 2 g fat (0 g saturated) | 13 g sugar
2.6 g fiber | 153 mg sodium

Though its packaging is free of cartoon characters, this fiber-void disaster is worse than most junk cereals.

Quaker Life

160 calories | 2 g fat (0 g saturated) | 8 g sugar
2.5 g fiber | 213 mg sodium

Life isn't the worst cereal on the shelf, but it does pack in more than three times as much sugar as fiber.

General Mills Cinnamon Chex

160 calories | 2.6 g fat (0 g saturated) | 11 g sugar
1.3 g fiber | 240 mg sodium

This cereal delivers more than 130 calories of pure carbohydrates.

Kellogg's Smart Start Strong Heart Original Antioxidants

190 calories | 1 g fat (0 g saturated) | 14 g sugar
3 g fiber | 200 mg sodium

What's so smart about a high-sugar, low-fiber cereal?
We still don't know.

Health Valley Organic Oat Bran Flakes

190 calories | 1.5 g fat (0.5 g saturated) | 11 g sugar
4 g fiber | 190 mg sodium

Sugar outnumbers fiber nearly three to one, which practically
guarantees you'll be hungry just an hour after you finish your meal.

Bear Naked Go Bananas . . . Go Nuts Granola (½ cup)

280 calories | 14 g fat (4 g saturated) | 10 g sugar
4 g fiber | 10 mg sodium

Granola may be the most overrated breakfast food of all time.
What do you think is holding all those banana-y clumps together?
Sugar and oil. And 4 grams of fiber just isn't enough to save
this bowl.

Quaker Real Medleys Apple Walnut Oatmeal (1 container)

290 calories | 8 g fat (1 g saturated) | 22 g sugar
5 g fiber | 270 mg sodium

A full 30 percent of these calories come from sugar.

Kellogg's Cracklin' Oat Bran

267 calories | 9 g fat (4 g saturated) | 19 g sugar
8 g fiber | 180 mg sodium

Nearly 20 grams of sugar alone make this cereal less than
wholesome, but Cracklin' Oat Bran also comes with a dose of
palm oil, which suppresses your appetite-control hormones.

Quaker Natural Granola Oats, Honey & Almonds

400 calories | 12 g fat (1 g saturated) | 20 g sugar
10 fiber | 50 mg sodium

Rumors of granola's healthfulness have been vastly overstated. Most brands are high in both sugar and total calories.

Quaker Cinnamon Oatmeal Squares with Cinnamon

210 calories | 2.5 g fat (0.5 g saturated) | 9 g sugar
5 g fiber | 190 mg sodium

This "healthy" cereal is overloaded with cheap refined carbs like maltodextrin.

Cascadian Farms Cinnamon Raisin Granola (⅔ cup)

230 calories | 3 g fat (0.5 g saturated) | 18 g sugar
3 g fiber | 230 mg sodium

Sugar is the second ingredient, followed closely by honey, molasses, and malted barley extract.

chapter # 9

ZERO SUGAR LUNCHES

EVER SEE THOSE NATURE PROGRAMS where the innocent herbivore herds are forced to gather at the watering hole, ever aware that crocodiles lurk below and lions watch from the bushes? That's sort of what lunchtime is to modern humans—at least, when it comes to our weight-loss plans.

That's because for most of us, a combination of stress, indecision, and time constraints often collide in a midday maelstrom of bad choices. A healthy Zero Sugar breakfast is easy to grab at home; dinner—even if it's eaten out—at least affords us the luxury of studying the offerings and asking a few questions. But lunch? Oftentimes you're standing in line, squinting to see the menu board while antsy, impatient, "I'm more important than you" types are tapping their toes behind you.

And much of what's on offer for lunch, be it at the nearest takeout place, the office vending machine, or wherever the gang is going on their break, isn't particularly good for you. One study found that just having a lot of take-out options near your work or along your commute to work makes you twice as likely to be obese. Think about that for a moment: Just the mere presence of take-out food increases your risk of obesity.

Your best bet is a Zero Sugar lunch you bring from home and quickly whip up in the office kitchenette. I've included plenty of them here. But if you just have to get out for lunch more often than not, there are still plenty of smart options available that fall within the Zero Sugar guidelines.

MAXIMIZE YOUR LUNCH

Get 100 Percent: There Are Good Breads

There are bad breads. There may even be well-meaning but stupid breads. But more and more, there are bad breads being disguised as good breads. "Wheat" breads, "multi-grain" breads, "7/9/12 grain" breads—they all offer the promise of whole-grain goodness, but often the reality is so much less than what's advertised. Many restaurants (such as Panera) make their "whole wheat" bread with mostly white flour. Look for the words "100% whole grain" when selecting an armature for your sandwich. And make sure there is no added sugar.

Load Up on Vegetables

Breakfast is fruit time. Dinner is, often, starch time. Make lunch vegetable time—opt for a salad, pile that sandwich high with produce, or look for other ways to get greens into your midday meal.

Pair Protein, Fiber, and Healthy Fat

Lunch has a job, and that job is to tide you over until dinner without your getting so ravenously hungry that you stop for a slice of pepperoni pizza on your way home. Protein, fiber, and healthy fat are the three hunger quenchers to look for: a salad with olive oil and vinegar (none of that fat-free stuff) and a protein source like turkey or nuts will help keep your belly from rumbling.

Don't Lose the Epic Wrap Battle

Those paper-thin wraps that seem so much healthier than bread are almost always loaded with calories, thanks to the fat that's needed to make them pliable—a large wrap can be the carb and calorie equivalent of four or five slices of bread.

Make an Upside-Down Salad

This genius idea was pioneered by Jason Lawless, once the executive chef at White Street restaurant in Tribeca. To build a salad that you can bring from home without it getting soggy, put the dressing at the bottom of a mason jar, and then add protein (like chicken, cheese, salmon chunks, or turkey slices). After that, add your larger veggies (such as tomatoes or peppers), and then top with greens. Seal the jar and, when you're ready to eat, simply turn it upside down on a plate.

Snack After Lunch, Not Before

A study published in the *Journal of the American Dietetic Association* found that mid-morning snackers tend to eat more throughout the day than afternoon snackers. Researchers found that dieters with the mid-morning munchies lost an average of 7 percent of their total body weight while those who did not snack before lunch lost more than 11 percent of their body weight. That's a difference of nearly 6.5 pounds for a 160-pound woman with a weight-loss goal. Moreover, afternoon snacking was associated with a slightly higher intake of fruits and vegetables.

Stick to Your Favorites

There's nothing wrong with settling on a handful of go-to lunches and eating the same nutritious thing every day. A 2015 study at the Friedman School of Nutrition Science and Policy at Tufts University looked at the diets of 6,814 people and found that the more diverse a person's diet, the more likely she was to experience weight gain. In fact, those who ate the widest range of foods showed a 120 percent greater increase in waist circumference compared with those who had the least diversity. In other words, people who have the best success at weight loss pick a set number of foods and tend to stick to them.

Beware the Celebrities

Signature sandwiches or those named after sports or movie stars are typically loaded with more cheap cheese than a celebrity memoir. Whenever you can, build your own sandwich so you can control the nutritional contents.

Custom-Build Your Greens

Approach a salad the way Donald Trump approaches a golf course: Build it the way you want it, no matter what anyone else says. Many ready-to-eat salads at sandwich or convenience shops are comprised of low-quality meats basking in oil and resting atop a field of wilted iceberg lettuce. Instead, customize your salad with high-quality greens like kale, spinach, or romaine lettuce; plenty of colorful vegetables; and high-quality proteins like nuts and grilled chicken.

Watch the Salt

One recent British study found that for every additional 1,000 milligrams of sodium you eat a day, your risk of obesity spikes by 25 percent. Yet keeping your sodium intake under the maximum daily allotment of 2,300 milligrams can be challenging when every single burger at a lunch spot like Chili's clocks in at more than 3,200 milligrams.

Don't Let This Dressing Make You Look Fat

There's not a traditional salad dressing recipe in the whole world that calls for sugar as part of the mix. But the vast majority of commercially available dressings—from the bottles you buy at the supermarket to the stuff on offer at your local restaurant—are loaded with it. Consider packing your own homemade version, or cut the normal amount of dressing in half to cut down on the added sugars.

Keep It Simple

If you are hitting a burger joint, most fast-food restaurants will actually offer lower-calorie fare than their sit-down counterparts. But as a rule, burgers with shorter and more simple names are better choices than those with protracted names. Upgrading from a bacon cheeseburger to an A.1. Ultimate Bacon Cheeseburger at Burger King, for example, will cost you an additional 520 calories.

Stay Chill

When you're ordering a sandwich, that is. Thanks to sauces, melted cheese, and lots of greasy meat, hot sandwiches are usually higher in fat and calories than cold sandwiches.

Have Breakfast for Lunch

As I surveyed the restaurant landscape, I found a lot of places—from McDonald's to IHOP—that offered nothing on their lunch menus that adhered to the Zero Sugar guidelines. The good news: Thanks to the recent "breakfast wars" between fast-food restaurants, many places now offer breakfast all day long. If you can't find anything on the menu that fits, don't be shy about ordering up an omelet or one of the recommended breakfasts from chapter 6.

PACK-AT-HOME LUNCHES

Big Salmon Salad

4 cups romaine lettuce

+ ½ medium cucumber, chopped

+ ½ cup cherry tomatoes

+ ½ cup cooked wheat berries

+ 4 oz Bumble Bee salmon pouch

+ 2 tsp chopped parsley

+ 1 Tbsp extra-virgin olive oil

+ lemon juice

> 399 calories | 17.2 g fat (2.2 g saturated) | 5.9 g natural sugar
> 3.4 g fiber | 34.5 g protein | 380 mg sodium

Southwestern Quinoa Salad

1 cup cooked quinoa

+ ½ cup black beans

+ ¼ cup defrosted frozen corn

+ 1 tsp extra-virgin olive oil

+ 1 Tbsp lime juice

+ 2 Tbsp chopped cilantro

+ pinch of cayenne pepper

> 405 calories | 8.5 g fat (1 g saturated) | 3 g natural sugar
> 14 g fiber | 16 g protein | 475 mg sodium

Tofu Fo' U

5 Boston lettuce leaves

+ ½ red bell pepper, thinly sliced

+ 2 pieces sesame ginger Nasoya Tofu (baked)

+ ¼ cup sliced almonds

+ thinly sliced scallion

+ 1 Tbsp sesame seeds

> 393 calories | 26 g fat (3.5 g saturated) | 6.2 g natural sugar
> 8 g fiber | 24 g protein | 407 mg sodium

Hummus Picnic

Single serving Sabra hummus

+ 2 Triscuits

+ ½ orange bell pepper, sliced

+ 2 stalks celery, sliced

+ 1 single serving olives

+ 100 calorie pack Emerald Nuts

> 265 calories | 18.5 g fat (2.2 g saturated) | 4 g natural sugar
> 7.8 g fiber | 6.8 g protein | 410 mg sodium

Turkey Tortilla

1 Ezekiel 4:9 whole-grain tortilla

+ 3 oz deli turkey

+ 1 tsp horseradish sauce

+ 2 romaine lettuce leaves

+ side of 1 cup grape tomatoes

> 300 calories | 7.5 g fat (1 g saturated) | 7.5 g natural sugar
> 8 g fiber | 26 g protein | 847 mg sodium

Unhurried Curried Salad

3 oz rotisserie chicken

+ 1 tsp mayonnaise

+ 2 Tbsp chopped celery

+ 5 red grapes, halved

+ ½ tsp curry powder

Serve on top of 3 cups salad greens.

+ ½ cup cooked quinoa, and sprinkle with 2 Tbsp slivered almonds

> 368 calories | 13 g fat (1.5 g saturated) | 8 g natural sugar
> 8 g fiber | 33 g protein | 336 mg sodium

ON-THE-GO LUNCHES (after the first fourteen days)

Fast Food

Taco Bell

Fresco Soft Taco—shredded chicken (order 2)

> 280 calories | 7 g fat (2 g saturated) | 4 g sugar
> 4 g fiber | 20 g protein | 940 mg sodium

order with: **Black beans**

> 80 calories | 1.5 fat (0 g saturated) | 1 g sugar
> 5 g fiber | 4 g protein | 200 mg sodium

Fresco Bean Burrito

> 350 calories | 9 g fat (2.5 g saturated) | 4 g sugar
> 9 g fiber | 13 g protein | 1,040 mg sodium

Fresco Burrito Supreme—chicken

> 340 calories | 8 g fat (2.5 g saturated) | 4 g sugar
> 6 g fiber | 19 g protein | 1,060 mg sodium

Add to any meal: Unlimited hot sauce packets

Burger King

Chicken Caesar Garden Fresh Salad Wrap (grilled)

340 calories | 16 g fat (3.5 g saturated) | 3 g sugar
4 g fiber | 21 g protein | 960 mg sodium

Wendy's

Power Mediterranean Chicken Salad
(hold the dressing, double the hummus—you'll save 10 grams of sugar!)

380 calories | 13 g fat (3.5 g saturated) | 8 g sugar
8 g fiber | 40 g protein | 1,020 mg sodium

Rich & Meaty Chili (small)

170 calories | 5 g fat (2 g saturated) | 6 g sugar
4 g fiber | 15 g protein | 780 mg sodium

order with: **Baked potato with broccoli** (no cheese; eat half)

300 calories | 0.5 g fat (0 g saturated) | 4 g sugar
9 g fiber | 10 g protein | 45 mg sodium

Diners

Denny's

Fit Fare Alaska Salmon

520 calories | 15 g fat (4 g saturated) | 3 g sugar
6 g fiber | 39 g protein | 1,260 mg sodium

Bob Evans

Farm Festival Bean Soup (bowl)

220 calories | 4.5 g fat (2 g saturated) | 2 g sugar
11 g fiber | 11 g protein | 1,030 mg sodium

Sandwich and Wrap Shops

Subway

6″ Veggie Delite (9-grain wheat bread, cucumbers, green peppers, lettuce, red onions, tomatoes, vinegar, avocado)

203 calories | 8 g fat (1.5 g saturated) | 6 g sugar
8 g fiber | 9 g protein | 280 mg sodium

6" Turkey Breast (9-grain wheat bread, cucumbers, green peppers, lettuce, red onions, tomatoes, mustard, avocado)

> 262 calories | 9 g fat (1.5 g saturated) | 7 g sugar
> 8 g fiber | 18 g protein | 780 mg sodium

Chipotle Chicken with Guacamole Salad (no dressing)

> 520 calories | 40 g fat (9 g saturated) | 6 g sugar
> 8 g fiber | 24 g protein | 880 mg sodium

Turkey and Guacamole Bacon Salad (hold the bacon; no dressing)

> 255 calories | 14.5 g fat (2 g saturated) | 5 g sugar
> 8 g fiber | 14 g protein | 650 mg sodium

Black Bean Soup (bowl)

> 210 calories | 1 g fat (0 g saturated) | 6 g sugar
> 15 g fiber | 12 g protein | 860 mg sodium

Panera Bread

Turkey Chili (bowl)

> 320 calories | 11 g fat (2 g saturated) | 7 g sugar
> 12 g fiber | 17 g protein | 1,090 mg sodium

Black Bean Soup (bowl)

> 230 calories | 3.5 g fat (0.5 g saturated) | 2 g sugar
> 9 g fiber | 17 g protein | 1,120 mg sodium

Mediterranean Chicken and Quinoa Salad

> 580 calories | 38 g fat (6 g saturated) | 4 g sugar
> 8 g fiber | 25 g protein | 870 mg

Lentil Quinoa Bowl (with chicken or egg)

> 390 calories | 8 g fat (1.5 g saturated) | 6 g sugar
> 10 g fiber | 34 g protein | 1,390 mg sodium

Cosí

Adobo Chicken with Avocado Bowl

> 473 calories | 18 g fat (4 g saturated) | 6 g sugar
> 10 g fiber | 24 g protein | 1,000 mg sodium

Chipotle

Salad Bowl with black beans, fajita vegetables, tomato salsa, and guacamole

> 400 calories | 23.5 g fat (3.5 g saturated) | 8 g sugar
> 21 g fiber | 12 g protein | 1,015 mg sodium

Salad bowl with chicken, pinto beans, fajita vegetables, and roasted chili-corn salsa

> 405 calories | 10 g fat (3 g saturated) | 8 g sugar
> 15.5 g fiber | 43 g protein | 1,080 mg sodium

Soft corn tacos with tofu sofritas, fajita vegetables, tomatillo green-chili salsa, and romaine lettuce

> 395 calories | 10.5 g fat (1.5 g saturated) | 8 g sugar
> 11.5 g fiber | 12 g protein | 1,010 mg sodium

Crispy corn tacos with chicken, black beans, fresh tomato salsa, and romaine lettuce

> 535 calories | 15.5 g fat (6 g saturated) | 4.5 g sugar
> 20.5 g fiber | 43 g protein | 810 mg sodium

Burrito bowl with brown rice, pinto beans, fajita vegetables, and tomatillo red chili salsa

> 375 calories | 7 g fat (1 g saturated) | 3 g sugar
> 15 g fiber | 11 g protein | 1,165 mg sodium

Coffee Shops

Starbucks

Hearty veggie and brown rice salad bowl

> 430 calories | 22 g fat (3 g saturated) | 8 g sugar
> 8 g fiber | 10 g protein | 640 mg sodium

Au Bon Pain

Southwest chicken salad

> 390 calories | 16 g fat (2.5 g saturated) | 10 g sugar
> 12 g fiber | 31 g protein | 730 mg sodium

Barley and creamy lentil soup, large

280 calories | 5 g fat (0.5 g saturated) | 4 g sugar
9 g fiber | 12 g protein | 930 mg sodium

Black bean soup, large

360 calories | 2 g fat (0 g saturated) | 4 g sugar
37 g fiber | 22 g protein | 1,420 mg sodium

Curried rice and lentil soup, large

240 calories | 1 g fat (0 g saturated) | 6 g sugar
11 g fiber | 12 g protein | 1,420 mg sodium

French Moroccan tomato lentil soup, large

260 calories | 3 g fat (0 g saturated) | 8 g sugar
17 g fiber | 13 g protein | 1,430 mg sodium

Swiss chard and three-bean soup, large

270 calories | 6 g fat (1 g saturated) | 5 g sugar
13 g fiber | 10 g protein | 950 mg sodium

Tuscan white bean soup, large

310 calories | 6 g fat (0 g saturated) | 8 g sugar
21 g fiber | 15 g protein | 1,270 mg sodium

Vegetarian chili, large

340 calories | 2.5 g fat (0 g saturated) | 9 g sugar
32 g fiber | 19 g protein | 1,210 mg sodium

Turkey chili, large

450 calories | 12 g fat (2 g saturated) | 7 g sugar
22 g fiber | 26 g protein | 1,090 mg sodium

Sit-Down Chains

Olive Garden

Herb grilled salmon

460 calories | 28 g fat (8 g saturated) | 3 g sugar
4 g fiber | 43 g protein | 570 mg sodium

order with: Double side of steamed broccoli

40 calories | 0 g fat | 4 g sugar
4 g fiber | 4 g protein | 40 mg sodium

Baked tilapia with shrimp

360 calories | 12 g fat (6 g saturated) | 4 g sugar
5 g fiber | 52 g protein | 1,130 mg sodium

order with: Double side of steamed broccoli

60 calories | 0 g fat | 3 g sugar
5 g fiber | 5 g protein | 60 mg sodium

TGI Fridays

Blackened Ahi Tuna Cobb Salad (full)

550 calories | 37 g fat (0 g saturated) | 9 g sugar
9 g fiber | 41 g protein | 1,160 mg sodium

Pecan crusted chicken salad (lunch-size)

540 calories | 36 g fat (8 g saturated) | 15 g sugar
6 g fiber | 20 g protein | 970 mg sodium

order with: Fresh broccoli

50 calories | 0.5 g fat (0 g saturated) | 0 g sugar
5 g fiber | 3 g protein | 370 mg sodium

Chipotle Yucatan Chicken Salad (lunch-size)

400 calories | 27 g fat (8 g saturated) | 11 g sugar
6 g fiber | 22 g protein | 710 mg sodium

order with: Fresh broccoli

50 calories | 0.5 g fat (0 g saturated) | 0 g sugar
5 g fiber | 3 g protein | 370 mg sodium

Chili's

Black bean burger, no bun

190 calories | 7 g fat (1 g saturated) | 2 g sugar
17 g fiber | 8 g protein | 540 mg sodium

order with: Asparagus and garlic roasted tomatoes

70 calories | 1.5 g fat (0 g saturated) | 4 g sugar
4 g fiber | 4 g protein | 410 mg sodium

chapter

10

ZERO SUGAR SNACKS

YOU ARE THE MODEL OF STEELY DISCIPLINE. A cold-eyed warrior unfazed by midday munchies, by late-night longings, by the siren song of Cinnabon. You stick to your three squares, restrict calories, and never allow yourself a salacious snack.

Congratulations. You've made weight loss an awful lot harder than it ought to be.

Here's the problem: Resisting snacks, restricting calories, being "disciplined"? Sadly, that very ascetic approach to eating makes it more difficult to keep your metabolism revving. When your snacking is lacking, so, too, is your body's ability to burn fat—the key to long-term leanness. In fact, those who eat at least six times a day have lower body-mass indexes, and consume fewer calories overall, than those who limit themselves to three squares, according to a 2015 study in the *Journal of the Academy of Nutrition and Dietetics*.

But that doesn't mean you should tear open the nearest bag of Cheetos and dive in. The snack aisle of your local supermarket is strewn with questionable chemicals, catastrophic calories, and snacks that are stripped of all their sustenance. Making the smart choice is critical.

MAXIMIZE YOUR SNACKS

Watch the Clock

Having a bite to hold you over 'til lunch is common practice, but a study published in the *Journal of the American Dietetic Association* found that mid-morning snackers tended to snack more throughout the day than afternoon snackers, resulting in hindered weight-loss efforts. Afternoon snacking was associated with a slightly higher intake of fiber and fruits and vegetables.

Color Code Your Snacks

You can avoid a mindless binge by adding visual traffic lights to your snack. Researchers at the University of Pennsylvania and Cornell University gave one set of students a bowl of uniform yellow chips, while another group had their regular snack layered with differently colored chips. Students who had their snack segmented ate 50 percent less than those with a uniform bowl.

Muscle Up Your Munchies

Make sure your snack contains protein, which requires more energy to burn than carbs or fats and thus keeps you fuller longer. But don't take it from me: In a study in the journal *Appetite*, researchers from the University of Missouri compared the satiety effects of high-, moderate-, and low-protein yogurts on twenty-four- to twenty-eight-year-old women, and found Greek yogurt, with the highest protein content, to have the greatest effect.

Beware, Costco Shoppers

A 2015 study in the journal *Appetite* found that the larger the bottle, bag, or box the food comes in, the larger we think the serving size should be. Researchers surveyed more than thirteen thousand people and found that when confronted with larger packages of cola, chips, chocolate, or lasagna, the shoppers tended to want to serve themselves larger portions.

Swap Hands

Want to snack less without going snackless? Try the left-handed diet (assuming you're right-handed . . .). Research in *Personality and Social Psychology Bulletin* found moviegoers grabbed for less popcorn when doing so with their nondominant hand. Eating with your nondominant hand makes you think about what you're doing and may help you eat less.

Use Smaller Bowls

Grabbing handfuls from the bag is never a good idea, but munching from a punch bowl won't do much for weight loss either. A study in *The FASEB Journal* suggests that overeating may be associated with the size of our serveware. Participants who were given larger bowls served and ate 16 percent more than those given smaller bowls. Not only that, the big-bowlers underestimated just how much they were eating by 7 percent! Take advantage of the visual illusion with belly-friendly bowls or ramekins.

Don't Be Duped

Just because something is marketed as "low fat" doesn't mean it's good for you—or you should eat more of it. A Cornell University study printed in the *Journal of Marketing Research* suggests people eat more of a snack that's marketed as "low fat." Participants in the study ate a whopping 28 percent more of a snack (M&M'S!) labeled "low fat" than when they didn't have the label.

MAKE-AT-HOME SNACKS

The Perfect Cracker Snacker

High-fiber crackers that aren't packed with added sugar can be hard
to come by. But they're out there: half a dozen Triscuits, for example,
gives you 3 grams of fiber and zero sugar. But for the ultimate cracker
snack, I love GG Bran Crispbread.

GG Bran Crispbread, 2 crackers

50 calories | 1 g fat (0 g saturated) | 0 g natural sugar
8 g fiber | 3 g protein | 80 mg sodium

Pair with:

▶ Almond butter

1 tablespoon: 98 calories | 9 g fat (1 g saturated) | 4.5 g natural sugar
10 g fiber | 21 g protein | 7 mg sodium

▶ Peanut butter

1 tablespoon (natural—no sugar added):
94 calories | 8 g fat (1 g saturated) | 1 g natural sugar
1 g fiber | 4 g protein | 78 mg sodium

▶ Hummus

2 Tbsp: 50 calories | 3 g fat (0.5 g saturated) | 0 g natural sugar
2 g fiber | 2.5 g protein | 114 mg sodium

▶ Avocado

¼: 80 calories | 7 g fat (1 g saturated) | 0 g natural sugar
3.5 g fiber | 1 g protein | 4 mg sodium

▶ Wholly Guacamole 100 calorie pack

100 calories | 9 g fat (1.5 g saturated) | 0 g natural sugar
3 g fiber | 1 g protein | 200 mg sodium

▶ Turkey breast

2 slices: 30 calories | 1 g fat (0 g saturated) | 1 g natural sugar
0 g fiber | 11 g protein | 277 mg sodium

▶ Smoked salmon

1 ounce: 33 calories | 1 g fat (0 g saturated) | 0 g natural sugar
0 g fiber | 5 g protein | 567 mg sodium

The Path Finder

This take on trail mix uses bran cereal to max out the fiber and keep you full all afternoon.

Post Shredded Wheat Original Spoon Size, ½ cup

85 calories | 1 g fat (0 g saturated) | 0 g sugar
13 g fiber | 3 g protein | 0 mg sodium

Mix with:

▶ Peanuts

2 Tbsp: 160 calories | 14 g fat (3 g saturated) | 1 g natural sugar
3 g fiber | 7 g protein | 0 g sodium

▶ Sliced almonds

¼ cup: 133 calories | 11.5 g fat (1 g saturated) | 1 g natural sugar
3 g fiber | 5 g protein | 0 g sodium

▶ Cashews

2 Tbsp: 163 calories | 13 g fat (2.5 g saturated) | 1.5 g natural sugar
9 g fiber | 181 mg sodium

▶ Shredded unsweetened coconut

3 Tbsp: 100 calories | 10 g fat (9 g saturated) | 1 g natural sugar
2 g fiber | 1 g protein | 5 mg sodium

▶ Sunflower seeds

1 Tbsp: 102 calories | 9 g fat (1 g saturated) | 0.5 g natural sugar
1.5 g fiber | 3.5 g protein | 2 mg sodium

▶ Unlimited spices: Curry powder, chili powder, smoked paprika, cinnamon, pumpkin pie spice, nutmeg, and more.

The Pop Star

In theory, popcorn is a terrific low-calorie, high-fiber snack. In reality, though, the popcorn in your bowl can be as scary as the movie you're watching while you eat it. Most microwave popcorn packages, for example, are lined with perfluorooctanoic acid (PFOA), which is also used to make Teflon products. PFOA can seep into the popcorn during the microwaving process, and it's been linked to infertility and weight gain, as well as impaired learning. And if your popcorn is butter-flavored, it's probably got a nice helping of diacetyl, a chemical that has been shown to break down the protective cell layers of the brain.

Instead of mind-altering microwave popcorn, opt for air-popped varieties and avoid the salt and fat overload by playing with a range of healthy spices.

Air-popped popcorn, 4 cups (season with herbs and spices like oregano and lemon zest, or ground chipotle)

> 124 calories | 1.5 g fat (0 g saturated) | 0 g sugar
> 5 g fiber | 4 g protein | 3 mg sodium

GRAB-AND-GO SNACKS

The Good Bean chickpea snacks, sea salt or cracked pepper, 1 oz

> 120 calories | 3 g fat (0 g saturated) | 1 g natural sugar
> 5 g fiber | 5 g protein | 185 mg sodium

Biena Snacks chickpea snacks, sea salt or habanero, ¼ cup

> 120 calories | 3 g fat (0 g saturated) | 0 g natural sugar
> 6 g fiber | 6 g protein | 260 mg sodium

Pulse Roasted Chickpeas chickpea snacks, original, spicy lemon zest, or sea salt and garlic, 1 oz

> 110 calories | 2 g fat (0 g saturated) | 3 g natural sugar
> 5 g fiber | 5 g protein | 115 mg sodium

KIND bar, Madagascar almond vanilla

> 210 calories | 16 g fat (1.5 g saturated) | 4 g natural sugar
> 6 g fiber | 7 g protein | 15 mg sodium

Qi'a Superfoods hot oatmeal, creamy coconut, cinnamon pumpkin seed, or superseeds and grains, 1 packet

> 160 calories | 6 g fat (4 g saturated) | 1 g natural sugar
> 5 g fiber | 6 g protein | 0 mg sodium

Quaker Instant Oatmeal (original flavor), 1 packet

> 100 calories | 2 g fat (0 g saturated) | 0 g natural sugar
> 3 g fiber | 4 g protein | 75 mg sodium

Note: It's very easy for oatmeal to go from healthy breakfast to tooth-rattling dessert. Quaker's Strawberries and Cream Instant Oatmeal packs 12 grams of sugar—six times as much sugar as fiber. Always opt for unflavored oatmeal and add your own fruit and spices.

Fruits and vegetables (not dried, or blended in a smoothie): Unlimited

Zero Sugar all-star choices:

Blackberries, 1 cup

> 62 calories | 1 g fat (0 g saturated) | 7 g natural sugar
> 7.5 g fiber | 2 g protein | 1 mg sodium

Raspberries, 1 cup

> 64 calories | 1 g fat (0 g saturated) | 5.5 g natural sugar
> 8 g fiber | 1.5 g protein | 1 mg sodium

Jicama, 1 cup slices

> 46 calories | 0 g fat | 2 g natural sugar
> 6 g fiber | 1 g protein | 5 mg sodium

Edamame, ¾ cup boiled

> 141 calories | 6 g fat (1 g saturated) | 2.5 g natural sugar
> 6 g fiber | 14 g protein | 7 mg sodium

chapter

11

ZERO SUGAR DINNERS

DINNER IS THE BIG FINALE of any day's eating and, in a lot of ways, it's the meal that defines us. The people we share dinner with are the people who matter most to us; the places we eat are the places that we most relate to. Dinner puts your whole day's food experience into perspective.

And for most Americans, dinner is where the majority of our protein is found. An egg squeezed between two English muffin halves or a few shavings of turkey stuffed into a sandwich isn't the same as a nice pot roast, a juicy burger, or a chicken dinner. In fact, the average American gets three times as much protein at dinner as he or she does at breakfast.

But that's a mistake. Eating protein throughout the day, rather than as a centerpiece for dinner, is better for keeping your muscles strong, according to a 2014 study in *The Journal of Nutrition*. The researchers found that a moderate amount of protein three times a day was more effective at stimulating muscle protein synthesis (i.e., the process of building lean, fat-burning muscle tissue) than relying on the evening meal for the majority of your meat.

What that means for you is that dinner shouldn't look like a hunk of meat with some starch on the side. While most traditional dinner foods are low in sugar—and, hence, fit easily into *Zero Sugar Diet*— your best approach is to keep your plate balanced more toward the vegetable arena.

And, because whole grains aren't as much of a player in traditional dinnertime fare, you may find hitting 8 grams of fiber at dinner to be a challenge—I did in trying to find heat-and-go dinners that worked. An easy answer: Simply have any of the grocery or restaurant foods listed in the lunch chapter for dinner instead.

MAXIMIZE YOUR DINNER

Don't Eat If You're Not Hungry

Ever get home late from the office, feeling pretty bedraggled and ready for bed, but you force yourself to eat dinner anyway? Don't do that. If you're not in the mood for your final meal, it's better to simply hit the hay and enjoy a nice breakfast the next day, according to a report from the *Journal of the Association for Consumer Research*. In a study of forty-five undergrads, researchers found that people who were moderately hungry before a meal tended to have lower blood glucose levels after eating than those who weren't particularly hungry before they ate.

Take the Scenic Route

If you've just sped through a stressful day at work, don't speed home. Stop at the playground and kick a ball with some kids, or swing by an art gallery, or meet a friend for tea. Prep yourself for dinner by finding a way to blow off the tensions of the day. Failing to let go of your work stress could lead to chronically elevated cortisol levels, causing sleep and immunity problems, blood-sugar abnormalities, and weight gain.

Pester Your Waiter

Chefs often add fat and salt to make meals taste better—but these ingredients aren't necessarily something they advertise on the menu. Since you've already taken such care to choose a dinner that sounds healthy, take the extra step and ask your server if there is any cream or butter in your dish. If there is, ask for your veggies and meats to be cooked dry and have sauces come on the side so you control how much ends up on your plate. No matter what kind of restaurant you're dining at, you can save up to 1,000 calories at each meal by making this simple request.

Picasso Up Your Plates

You know how dinner in a fancy restaurant comes served with a beautiful composition and a little sprig of parsley on the side? Do that at home, instead of just dumping everything on a platter and setting it out for the rabble to reach for. A study in the journal *Obesity* found that when food is served family-style, people consume 35 percent more over the course of the meal. When an additional helping requires leaving the table, people hesitate to go back for more.

Order Grown-up Drinks

A frozen margarita may sound refreshing, but most restaurants and bars have ditched their fresh-fruit recipes in favor of viscous syrups made mostly from high-fructose corn syrup and thickening agents. As a general rule, the more garnishes a drink has hanging from its rim, the worse it is for your waistline. Instead, choose a cocktail made with club soda and lime, or stick with nutrient-packed red wine.

Eat "Wet" Carbs

That doesn't mean soaking your potatoes in gravy. A wet carb is one that naturally has a lot of water in it—stuff like cucumbers, tomatoes, salad greens, and asparagus. Dry carbs, like bread, French fries, and pasta, require your body to give up water in order to digest them. Wet carbs, on the other hand, allow you to stay adequately hydrated overnight. That helps your body process the fiber you've eaten during the day and ensures you'll continue to draw nourishment from the day's food intake. Speaking of which,

Drink and Drink Again

Have a big tall glass of water before you go to bed, and set another on your nightstand.

Make Your Bed(time)

According to Wake Forest researchers, dieters who sleep five hours or less put on two and a half times more belly fat, while those who sleep more than eight hours pack on only slightly less than that. But when you have a regular bedtime and stick to it, you set yourself up for day-in, day-out weight loss. Shoot for an average of six to seven hours of sleep per night—the optimal amount for weight control.

MAKE-AT-HOME DINNERS

Wild at Heart Salmon

4 oz grilled wild salmon, with lemon juice

+ 4 cups baby spinach sautéed with garlic and 1 tsp extra-virgin olive oil

+ 1 cup diced potatoes cooked in 1 Tbsp sunflower oil

+ smoked Spanish paprika

+ 1 Tbsp crushed flaxseed

> 444 calories | 21 g fat (4 g saturated) | 2 g natural sugar
> 8.5 g fiber | 30 g protein | 148 mg sodium

Spice-Rubbed Chicken

1 Tbsp garlic powder

+ 1 Tbsp paprika, sprinkled on both sides of 1 4-oz chicken breast, grilled

+ 4 cups cauliflower florets, roasted with 1 Tbsp sunflower oil

423 calories | 24.5 g fat (3 g saturated) | 8 g natural sugar
8.5 g fiber | 34 g protein | 179 mg sodium

Sweet Potato Chickpea Bowl

Baked medium sweet potato (around 2"x5")

+ 2 cups baby spinach

+ ½ cup chickpeas

+ 2 Tbsp tahini blended with 1 Tbsp lemon juice

+ 2 Tbsp hot water

+ salt

+ garlic powder

429 calories | 18.6 g fat (2.5 g saturated) | 11.7 g natural sugar
14.1 g fiber | 16.4 g protein | 321 mg sodium

Mushroom Farrotto

1 cup cooked farro

+ 4 cups button mushrooms, sautéed with garlic and 1 tsp extra-virgin olive oil

+ ¼ cup canned white cannellini beans

+ 1 cup baby arugula

404 calories | 8 g fat (1 g saturated) | 8 g natural sugar
14 g fiber | 24 g protein | 247 mg sodium

Broccoli Pasta and Meatballs

4 cups broccoli slaw, sautéed

+ ½ cup Mario Batali marinara sauce

+ 6 cooked frozen Butterball turkey meatballs

+ 1 cup frozen peas, microwaved and added to mixture

> 420 calories | 16 g fat (4 g saturated) | 10 g natural sugar
> 8.5 g fiber | 22 g protein | 1,146 mg sodium

Tuna Burger

1 Whole Foods frozen yellowfin tuna burger

+ Ezekiel 4:9 sprouted whole-grain English muffin, toasted

+ 2 romaine lettuce leaves

+ 1 tomato slice

+ 1 red onion slice

+ 1 tsp olive oil–based mayo

+ a kale salad:

> 3 cups chopped kale
>
> + 1 tsp extra-virgin olive oil
>
> + lemon juice
>
> + 2 Tbsp sunflower seeds

> 417 calories | 22.8 g fat (2.8 g saturated) | 3 g natural sugar
> 8 g fiber | 31 g protein | 414 mg sodium

FROZEN DINNERS (after the first fourteen days)

Amy's Tortilla Casserole and Black Beans bowl

390 calories | 18 g fat (6 g saturated) | 6 g natural sugar
10 g fiber | 17 g protein | 780 mg sodium

Luvo Chicken Chipotle Chili

250 calories | 8 g fat (1 g saturated) | 7 g natural sugar
8 g fiber | 17 g protein | 490 mg sodium

Luvo Chicken Enchiladas

360 calories | 7 g fat (2 g saturated) | 7 g natural sugar
9 g fiber | 18 g protein | 420 mg sodium

Luvo Quinoa and Vegetable Enchiladas

370 calories | 8 g fat (2.5 g saturated) | 9 g natural sugar
10 g fiber | 13 g protein | 220 mg sodium

Tandoor Chef Vegetable Korma

330 calories | 11 g fat (2.5 g saturated) | 4 g natural sugar
8 g fiber | 10 g protein | 500 mg sodium

Tandoor Chef Kofta Curry with Channa Masala and Spinach Basmati Pilaf

400 calories | 19 g fat (3 g saturated) | 8 g natural sugar
9 g fiber | 10 g protein | 690 mg sodium

7 Days *of* Zero Sugar Recipes

These recipes can guide you through a week of Zero Sugar eating, or simply pull a few that look tempting and slip them into the other recommended meals in this book.

DAY 1 • BREAKFAST

Chocolate Vanilla Oatmeal

You'll need:

1 cup cooked oatmeal

1 tsp unsweetened cocoa powder

1 cup raspberries

½ tsp vanilla extract

What to do: Mix together and enjoy.

Nutrition:

227 calories | 6.1 g natural sugar | 12.4 g fiber | 4 g fat | 7.3 g protein

---

DAY 1 • LUNCH

Turkey Sandwich on Whole-Grain Bread

You'll need:

1 romaine lettuce leaf, cut in half

3 slices roast turkey

2 slices Cheddar cheese

2 slices 100% whole-grain sugar-free bread

2 tsp olive oil–based mayonnaise

What to do:

1. Make sure your bread delivers more fiber than sugar by checking the label. (I like Food for Life 7 Sprouted Grains.)
2. Pile high.

Nutrition per serving:

306 calories | 3 g natural sugar | 6 g fiber | 12.9 g fat | 19.3 g protein

DAY 1 • DINNER

Seared Ahi Tuna with Spinach Salad

You'll need:

3 Tbsp extra-virgin olive oil

1 Tbsp red wine vinegar

Salt, pepper, 1 Tbsp chopped fresh Italian herbs

5 oz ahi tuna steak

2 cups baby spinach

½ cup black beans

½ cup fresh peas

1 Tbsp chopped walnuts

1 Tbsp grated Parmesan cheese

What to do:

1. Make the dressing: Combine 2 Tbsp olive oil, the vinegar, dash of salt and pepper, and herbs.

2. Heat the remaining 1 Tbsp of oil in a pan over medium-high heat. Season the tuna with salt and pepper and place in the pan. Sear for 3 minutes on each side or to desired doneness.

3. Make the salad:

   a. Combine the spinach with the beans, peas, walnuts, and 2 Tbsp of the dressing.

   b. Top with Parmesan.

   Serve the tuna with the salad on the side.

Nutrition:

580 calories | 4.6 g natural sugar | 14.6 g fiber | 26.4 g fat | 18.2 g protein

BONUS: Enjoy with a glass (5 oz) of Rosé or Pinot Noir for an additional 122 calories.

DAY 1 • SNACK

Popcorn popped fresh in olive oil, lightly salted

(WOMEN: *1 cup,* MEN: *2 cups*)

Nutrition per 1-cup serving:

40 calories | 0 g natural sugar | 2 g fiber | 1.5 g fat | 1 g protein

---

Total daily nutrition:

WOMEN:
1,275 calories
16.3 g natural sugar
35.0 g fiber
44.8 g fat
45.8 g protein

MEN:
1,315 calories
16.3 g natural sugar
37.2 g fiber
46.3 g fat
46.8 g protein

DAY 2 • BREAKFAST

Burrito

You'll need:

1 egg, scrambled (MEN: 2 eggs)

½ cup black beans

2 Tbsp salsa

1 Tbsp shredded Cheddar cheese

1 Ezekiel wrap

What to do: Combine the egg, beans, salsa, and cheese onto the wrap.

Nutrition:
WOMEN: 283 calories | 3 g natural sugar | 10 g fiber | 9.8 g fat | 14.7 g protein
MEN: 353 calories | 3 g natural sugar | 10 g fiber | 14.8 g fat | 20.7 g protein

DAY 2 • LUNCH

Quinoa Salad

You'll need:

1 cup precooked quinoa

½ cup black beans, drained

¼ cup frozen corn kernels, defrosted

1 Tbsp chopped fresh cilantro

Pinch of cayenne pepper

1 tsp fresh lime juice

1 tsp extra-virgin olive oil

What to do:
1. Mix the quinoa, beans, corn, cilantro, and cayenne.
2. Dress with equal parts lime juice and olive oil.

Nutrition:
405 calories | 3 g natural sugar | 14 g fiber | 5.5 g fat | 12.3 g protein

DAY 2 • DINNER

Whole Wheat Pizza with Chicken and Asparagus

(makes 4 servings)

You'll need:

2 Tbsp extra-virgin olive oil

1 Tbsp grated Parmesan cheese

1 cup chopped asparagus

1 tsp Italian seasoning

¼ tsp dried red pepper flakes

Ready-made whole-grain flatbread pizza crust, 12 inches

1 cup sliced pear

¼ cup cooked chicken

1 cup part-skim shredded mozzarella cheese

What to do:

1. Preheat the oven to 425°F.
2. Mix 1 Tbsp olive oil with the Parmesan cheese and asparagus; arrange in a single layer on a rimmed baking sheet and roast in the oven for 10 minutes.
3. Combine the remaining 1 Tbsp olive oil with the Italian seasoning and red pepper flakes; brush over the pizza crust.
4. Spread the roasted asparagus, pear slices, and chicken evenly over the crust.
5. Sprinkle the mozzarella on top.
6. Place the pizza in the oven and bake for 7 to 10 minutes, or until the cheese is completely melted.

Nutrition per serving:

448 calories | 4 g natural sugar | 7.8 g fiber | 13.4 g fat | 16.2 g protein

BONUS: Enjoy with a glass (5 oz) of Gragnano wine for an additional 125 calories.

DAY 2 • SNACK

WOMEN:

Broccoli (1 cup)
with Hummus (2 Tbsp)

Nutrition:

80 calories | 1.5 g natural sugar | 3.3 g fiber | 2.8 g fat | 3.8 g protein

MEN:

Edamame (1 cup shelled)
with Hummus (1 Tbsp)

Nutrition:

225 calories | 2 g natural sugar | 9 g fiber | 7.4 g fat | 17.2 g protein

---

Total daily nutrition:

WOMEN:
1,341 calories
11.5 g natural sugar
35.1 g fiber
31.5 g fat
47 g protein

MEN:
1,556 calories
12 g natural sugar
40.8 g fiber
41.1 g fat
66.4 g protein

DAY 3 • BREAKFAST

Yogurt with Fruit and Nuts

You'll need:

½ cup blackberries

½ cup raspberries

¼ cup bran cereal

1 Tbsp sliced almonds

½ cup plain Greek yogurt

What to do: Mix the berries, bran, and almonds into the yogurt.

Nutrition:

231 calories | 12.8 g natural sugar | 13.7 g fiber | 8.5 g fat | 14.7 g protein

DAY 3 • LUNCH

Turkey Avocado Sandwich

You'll need:

2 tsp spicy mustard

2 slices sprouted grain bread

3 oz fresh roasted turkey breast (MEN: 5 oz)

½ cup avocado

1 cup arugula

What to do:

Spread the mustard on one slice of bread. Top with the turkey, avocado, arugula, and the second slice of bread.

Nutrition:

WOMEN:
449 calories | 1 g natural sugar | 11 g fiber | 15.3 g fat | 38.7 g protein
MEN:
553 calories | 1 g natural sugar | 11.4 g fiber | 19 g fat | 54.7 g protein

DAY 3 • DINNER

Pork Tenderloin with broccoli and cauliflower

(makes 2 servings)

You'll need:

2 Tbsp extra-virgin olive oil, plus more for coating the skillet

Salt and pepper

Minced garlic, for pork rub and for broccoli and cauliflower

Chopped fresh parsley

1 pound pork tenderloin

1 cup chopped broccoli

1 cup chopped cauliflower

1 Tbsp grated Parmesan cheese

MEN: add ¼ cup cooked lentils

What to do:

1. Preheat the oven to 400°F.
2. Combine 1 Tbsp olive oil with the salt, pepper, garlic, and parsley; rub onto the pork.
3. Coat an oven-proof skillet with olive oil and sear the pork on all sides.
4. Roast the pork in the oven for about 15 minutes, or until a meat thermometer reads 145°F to 150°F. Remove from the oven and let rest for 5 to 10 minutes.
5. Cut the pork into ½-inch-thick medallions.
6. Toss the chopped broccoli and cauliflower in the remaining 1 Tbsp olive oil and arrange in a single layer on a rimmed baking sheet; sprinkle with salt, pepper, garlic, and Parmesan.
7. Roast in the oven for 15 to 20 minutes, or until tender.
8. Serve the pork with broccoli and cauliflower (**MEN**: over lentils).

Nutrition per serving:

WOMEN:
380 calories | 1.8 g natural sugar | 2.2 g fiber | 13.2 g fat | 45.4 g protein
MEN:
438 calories | 5.4 g natural sugar | 7 g fiber | 14 g fat | 49.9 g protein

BONUS: Enjoy with a glass (5 oz) of Zinfandel for an additional 132 calories.

DAY 3 • SNACK

WOMEN:

Shelled Edamame (½ cup with dash of salt)

Nutrition:

100 calories | 1 g natural sugar | 4 g fiber | 3 g fat | 8 g protein

MEN:

Baked Tortilla Chips and Salsa

You'll need:

2 tsp avocado oil

1 whole wheat tortilla

2 Tbsp salsa

What to do:

1. Preheat the oven to 350°F.
2. Brush the avocado oil on both sides of the tortilla and cut it into wedges.
3. Bake for 5 to 6 minutes, turn over, and bake 4 to 5 minutes more.
4. Serve with salsa.

Nutrition:

231 calories | 0 g natural sugar | 5 g fiber | 12.8 g fat | 6 g protein

---

Total daily nutrition:

WOMEN:
1,292 calories
16.6 g natural sugar
30.9 g fiber
40.0 g fat
106.8 g protein

MEN:
1,585 calories
19.2 g natural sugar
37.1 g fiber
44.5 g fat
125.3 g protein

DAY 4 • BREAKFAST

Smoothie

You'll need:

¼ cup unsweetened almond milk

¼ cup silken tofu

2 kale leaves, stems removed

½ frozen banana

2 Tbsp chia seeds

1 ice cube (optional)

What to do:

1. Add the almond milk and tofu to the bowl of a blender.
2. Add the kale, banana, chia seeds, and ice cube, if desired. Blend until smooth.

Nutrition:

363 calories | 10 g natural sugar | 13 g fiber | 3 g fat | 6.3 g protein

DAY 4 • LUNCH

Shrimp, Mushroom, and Goat Cheese Flatbread

(makes 4 servings)

You'll need:

1 whole-grain flatbread, 12 inches

2 Tbsp extra-virgin olive oil

2 tsp Herbs de Provence

1 small red onion, sliced

2 cups white mushrooms, sliced

½ pound shrimp, peeled and deveined

1 cup baby spinach, coarsely chopped

½ cup roasted pumpkin seeds

2 oz goat cheese

What to do:

1. Brush the flatbread with 1 Tbsp olive oil and sprinkle evenly with the Herbs de Provence.
2. Heat the remaining 1 Tbsp oil in a sauté pan. Sauté the onion and mushrooms for 5 minutes, then add the shrimp and sauté until the shrimp are bright pink, cooking 2 to 3 minutes per side.
3. Arrange the spinach in a layer on the flatbread, then layer the mushroom, onions, and shrimp.
4. Top with the pumpkin seeds and goat cheese.

Nutrition per serving:

240 calories | 0.5 g natural sugar | 7.2 g fiber | 4.8 g fat | 16.3 g protein

DAY 4 • DINNER

Steak with Bulgur, Green Beans, and Asparagus

You'll need:

7 oz steak (such as strip or rib eye)

2 Tbsp walnut oil

Salt and pepper

1 cup fresh green beans, chopped

½ cup chopped fresh asparagus

2 Tbsp chopped walnuts

½ cup cooked bulgur

Fresh lemon juice

What to do:

1. Heat a grill to high.
2. Brush the steak with 1 Tbsp walnut oil and season with salt and pepper.
3. Arrange the green beans and asparagus on a double layer of aluminum foil, drizzle with the remaining 1 Tbsp oil, and season with salt and pepper; fold the foil to create a sealed packet.
4. Grill the steak over high heat, 6 to 8 minutes per side or to desired doneness; remove from the heat and let rest for 5 to 10 minutes.
5. Grill the foil packet for 10 to 15 minutes, or until the vegetables are tender.
6. Add the chopped walnuts to the vegetables and serve over bulgur. Squeeze fresh lemon juice to taste over the vegetables.
7. Serve with the steak.

Nutrition:

WOMEN: *3-oz serving:*
564 calories | 3.6 g natural sugar | 11 g fiber | 41.7 g fat | 27.3 g protein
MEN: *4-oz serving:*
680 calories | 3.6 g natural sugar | 11 g fiber | 52 g fat | 33.5 g protein

BONUS: Enjoy with a glass of Cabernet blend for an additional 120 calories.

DAY 4 • SNACK

Raspberry Almond Smoothie

You'll need:

1 cup raspberries

1 cup unsweetened almond milk

1 tsp unsweetened cocoa powder

Cup of ice

What to do:

Blend the ingredients and drink.

Nutrition:

98 calories | 5 g natural sugar | 9 g fiber | 3.3 g fat | 2.3 g protein

---

Total Daily Nutrition:

WOMEN:
1,385 calories
19.1 g natural sugar
40.2 g fiber
52.8 g fat
52.2 g protein

MEN:
1,501 calories
19.1 g natural sugar
40.2 g fiber
63.1 g fat
58.4 g protein

DAY 5 • BREAKFAST

Oatmeal with Berries and Almond Butter

You'll need:

½ cup raspberries

1 Tbsp almond butter

1 cup cooked oatmeal

What to do:

Combine the berries and almond butter into the oatmeal.

Nutrition:

285 calories | 5.6 g natural sugar | 11 g fiber | 20.4 g fat | 13.5 g protein

DAY 5 • LUNCH

Halibut Fish Sandwich

You'll need:

1 4-oz halibut fillet

2 tsp Dijon mustard

Salt and pepper

Fresh lemon juice

1 Tbsp olive oil mayonnaise

2 slices sprouted grain bread

Arugula

½ cup shredded fresh carrot

FOR MEN: 1 slice Cheddar cheese

FOR MEN: ½ cup edamame, shelled

What to do:

1. Preheat the oven to 400°F.
2. Rub the fish with the mustard and season with salt and pepper.
3. Bake the fish in the oven for 15 to 20 minutes, or until it flakes easily with a fork.
4. Squeeze the lemon juice over the baked fish.
5. Spread the mayo on the bread and build the sandwich with the fish, arugula, and carrot (and cheese for men).
6. **FOR MEN:** Serve edamame on the side.

Nutrition:

WOMEN:
380 calories | 5 g natural sugar | 7.5 g fiber | 6.5 g fat | 34.5 g protein
MEN:
593 calories | 6 g natural sugar | 11.5 g fiber | 18.5 g fat | 49.5 g protein

DAY 5 • DINNER

Chicken Kebabs

You'll need:

1 pound boneless chicken breast, cut into 1-inch cubes

½ cup all-natural teriyaki sauce

1 medium onion, cut into 1-inch pieces

1 bell pepper, cut into 1-inch pieces

2 zucchinis, cut into ½-inch-thick pieces

½ cup cooked quinoa

FOR MEN: ½ cup garbanzo beans

What to do:

1. Marinate the chicken cubes in teriyaki sauce for at least 30 minutes.
2. Divide the chicken, onion, bell pepper, and zucchini among 8 presoaked wooden skewers.
3. Brush with any remaining marinade.
4. Set a grill to medium heat, and grill the skewers for 6 to 7 minutes per side, or until cooked through.
5. Serve over quinoa (and garbanzo beans for men).

Nutrition (2 skewers):

WOMEN:
461 calories | 8.6 g natural sugar | 12.6 g fiber | 6 g fat | 39.9 g protein
MEN:
604 calories | 8.6 g natural sugar | 12.6 g fiber | 7.5 g fat | 46 g protein

BONUS: Enjoy with a glass (5 oz) of Sauvignon Blanc for an additional 120 calories.

DAY 5 • SNACK

Popcorn
(3 cups popped fresh in olive oil, lightly salted)

Nutrition:

120 calories | 0 g natural sugar | 6 g fiber | 4.5 g fat | 3 g protein

---

Total Daily Nutrition:

WOMEN:
1,366 calories
19.2 g natural sugar
37.1 g fiber
37.4 g fat
90.9 g protein

MEN:
1,722 calories
20.2 g natural sugar
41.1 g fiber
50.9 g fat
112.0 g protein

DAY 6 • BREAKFAST

Bran Cereal and Berries

You'll need:

½ cup no-sugar bran cereal

1 cup unsweetened almond milk

½ cup blackberries

What to do:

Eat the cereal with the almond milk; have the berries on the side.

Nutrition:

142 calories | 8.5 g natural sugar | 14 g fiber | 4 g fat | 5.5 g protein

DAY 6 • LUNCH

Beef Burger on Sprouted Grain Bread

Makes 4 servings

You'll need:

1 pound ground grass-fed beef (to make 4 patties)

1 medium onion, chopped

1 Tbsp extra-virgin olive oil

8 slices sprouted grain bread

Romaine lettuce

All natural organic horseradish mustard, 1 tsp per patty

1 medium tomato, cut into ½-inch slices

Fresh lemon juice

Salt, pepper, favorite seasonings

FOR MEN: 1 slice Cheddar cheese per burger

What to do:

1. Combine the ground beef with the onion and form into 4 patties. Season with salt and pepper.
2. Heat the olive oil in a skillet over medium heat.
3. Cook the patties for 4 to 6 minutes per side for medium-rare or until desired doneness.
4. Serve on bread with romaine lettuce leaves, mustard, and tomato (and cheese for men).

Nutrition using one patty:

WOMEN:
400 calories | 4.4 g natural sugar | 6.8 g fiber | 13.5 g fat | 31.5 g protein
MEN:
513 calories | 4.4 g natural sugar | 6.8 g fiber | 22.5 g fat | 38.5 g protein

DAY 6 • DINNER

Garlic and Butter Salmon with Beans

You'll need:

6 oz salmon fillet (wild caught, Pacific)

1 Tbsp all-natural butter, melted

Salt and pepper

2 cloves garlic, minced

¼ cup each of garbanzo, kidney, and black beans

1 Tbsp fresh lemon juice

Favorite seasonings

FOR MEN: ½ cup avocado slices

What to do:

1. Preheat the oven to 400°F.
2. Brush the salmon with the butter and season with salt, pepper, and garlic.
3. Bake in the oven for 15 to 20 minutes, until it flakes easily with a fork.
4. Combine the beans and add the lemon juice. Season to taste.
5. **WOMEN** get half the beans as a serving; **MEN** get the full portion.
6. Serve with the salmon (and avocado for men).

Nutrition:

WOMEN:
386 calories | 0.6 g natural sugar | 5.1 g fiber | 20.3 g fat | 33.1 g protein
MEN:
588 calories | 1.7 g natural sugar | 15.2 g fiber | 31 g fat | 40 g protein

BONUS: Enjoy with a glass (5 oz) of Pinot Noir for an additional 122 calories.

DAY 6 • SNACK

Edamame, 1 cup cooked, shelled

Nutrition:

200 calories | 2 g sugar | 8 g fiber | 6 g fat | 16 g protein

---

Total Daily Nutrition:

WOMEN:
1,250 calories
15.5 g natural sugar
33.9 g fiber
43.8 g fat
86.1 g protein

MEN:
1,565 calories
16.6 g natural sugar
44 g fiber
63.5 g fat
100 g protein

DAY 7 • BREAKFAST

Oatmeal with Berries

You'll need:

1 cup cooked oatmeal

½ cup raspberries

1 tsp vanilla extract

FOR MEN: 2 Tbsp raw almond butter

What to do:

Combine all of the ingredients.

Nutrition:

WOMEN:
195 calories | 3.6 g natural sugar | 8 g fiber | 3.6 g fat | 6.5 g protein
MEN:
385 calories | 5.6 g natural sugar | 12 g fiber | 20.6 g fat | 13.5 g protein

DAY 7 • LUNCH

Steak Salad with Kale and Spinach

You'll need:

3-oz portion flank steak, grilled and cut into strips

1 cup baby kale

1 cup baby spinach

¼ cup chopped red onion

1 cup chopped carrots

¼ cup garbanzo beans

2 Tbsp balsamic vinegar

FOR MEN: ½ cup sweet peas

What to do:

Combine all of the ingredients and enjoy.

Nutrition:

WOMEN:
400 calories | 10 g natural sugar | 10 g fiber | 11.3 g fat | 28.7 g protein
MEN:
480 calories | 14 g natural sugar | 14 g fiber | 11.3 g fat | 32.7 g protein

DAY 7 • DINNER

Grilled Chicken and Lentils

You'll need:

5 oz chicken breast

2 Tbsp butter, melted (preferably all-natural made from milk of grass-fed cows)

Salt and pepper

1 tsp poultry seasoning

1 Tbsp extra-virgin olive oil

1 tsp each of minced garlic, rosemary, and thyme

1 Tbsp fresh lemon juice

½ cup cooked lentils

2 Tbsp feta cheese

¼ cup chopped cucumber

What to do:

1. Brush the chicken with 1 Tbsp of the melted butter. Season with salt, pepper, and poultry seasoning.
2. Grill the chicken over medium-high heat, about 6 minutes per side or until cooked through; remove from the heat and let rest for 5 minutes.
3. Combine the remaining Tbsp melted butter, olive oil, garlic, rosemary, thyme, and lemon juice. Mix into the cooked lentils, then add the feta and cucumber.
4. Cut the chicken into slices and serve over the lentils.

Nutrition:

476 calories | 3.3 g natural sugar | 7.8 g fiber | 28.3 g fat | 29.4 g protein

BONUS: Serve with a glass (5 oz) of Chardonnay for an additional 123 calories and about 1.4 g sugar.

DAY 7 • SNACK

WOMEN:

Popcorn (2 cups)

Nutrition:

80 calories | 0 g natural sugar | 4 g fiber | 3 g fat | 2 g protein

MEN:

Popcorn (3 cups)

Nutrition:

120 calories | 0 g natural sugar | 6 g fiber | 4.5 g fat | 3 g protein

---

Total Daily Nutrition:

WOMEN:
1,274 calories
16.9 g natural sugar
29.8 g fiber
46.2 g fat
66.6 g protein

MEN:
1,584 calories
22.9 g natural sugar
39.8 g fiber
64.7 g fat
78.6 g protein

chapter 12

THE SUGAR BURNER WORKOUTS

IMAGINE YOU'RE OUT FOR A WALK IN THE WOODS.

As you stroll along, you breathe in and out casually, enjoying the sweet natural air. Your body has access to plenty of oxygen, and so as you stroll along your muscles are primarily using a type of muscle fiber called slow-twitch fiber, which uses the oxygen you take in and circulates with every breath to burn off the glucose in your blood and the glycogen stored in your liver. Slow-twitch fibers are used in aerobic exercise and for anything that takes endurance, like this lovely little jaunt. At a leisurely pace, you're not even breathing hard, but you're burning off calories—all movement, even the blinking of your eyes, burns calories. If you walk at a brisk pace for an extended period of time—twenty minutes or more—you'll begin to run out of glucose. To replace that blood glucose, your body will begin to tap into your fat stores. But again, it will take quite some time for that to happen.

Suddenly, the path through the woods becomes a little steep and rocky. You keep right along with your pace, but your breath becomes a little bit labored, and there's a light burning sensation in your legs. You're beginning to expend energy at a higher rate, and your lungs are working overtime to supply oxygen to your muscles for them to burn. The glucose in your blood is being burned more quickly, too. But depending on how fit you are, there's a point at which the demand on your muscles outstrips what your lungs alone can meet. That's when you begin to tap into more of your fast-twitch muscle— the fibers that burn glycogen, the reserves of sugar stored in your muscles. Fast-twitch muscle is activated by high-intensity exercise like weight training or walking up steep hills. The burning sensation is caused by the waste products that are produced by your muscles when that sugar is burned. When we exercise aerobically, we train our bodies to develop more slow-twitch muscle, so we have more muscular endurance and can burn oxygen more efficiently. When we exercise anaerobically, we train our bodies to build more fast-twitch, sugar-burning muscle. Walking up a steep hill like this, you're actually doing a bit of both.

Now imagine you hear a crashing noise behind you. It's an enormous brown bear, out for blood, and you can see the stringy saliva dripping from its huge fangs. Suddenly you're sprinting as fast as you can, and even though you're fighting for as much air as you can get, it's primarily stored sugar that's propelling you up the hill. The muscles in your body are on fire as you burn glycogen like mad!

Just as you reach the peak, you catch a break: The bear gets distracted by a school of leaping salmon, and you collapse in a heap, finally safe. Depending on how recently you ate and how far you sprinted, your muscles probably feel like Jell-O, because you've burned all the sugar out of them. You might even feel dizzy because your blood sugar levels are so low.

As you rest and return to normal, your body starts to replace the missing glucose and glycogen by attacking your fat stores, turning them back into sugar to circulate through your blood and then convert into glycogen. It will also begin to go in search of calories to replenish your bloodstream and restore your muscles. The food you eat over the next several hours (you'll probably want a stiff drink, too) will go toward restoring your glycogen stores, but in the meantime, your body will start to break down fat to replace the needed sugar.

If you stop thinking about burning calories when you exercise, and start thinking about burning sugar, you'll begin to see why short, high-energy bursts of exercise make more sense. While long, slow workouts do indeed burn off sugar, the process takes quite a bit of time, and they don't really touch the extra sugar that's stored in your muscles. But when you do shorter, high-intensity workouts, you quickly burn off the stored sugar in your muscles, causing your body to melt down fat in order to replace the missing glycogen. And when you work out before a meal, you double your benefits; you not only cause your body to convert fat into sugar, but you create a big hole for all those delicious new calories to fall into, before they can be converted to fat.

The secret to getting around this seemingly impossible barrier: Exercise enough, but not too much. The exercise plan in this chapter —an optional part of *Zero Sugar Diet*—will make certain you do the ideal amount to help you lose your belly rapidly while greatly improving your fitness level.

Here's how it will happen: You will do a combination of brief workouts designed to burn less than 200 calories, including a full-body resistance-training workout that will put your high-protein diet to work building muscle and boosting your metabolism in ways that other exercise programs simply can't.

- ▶ Every day you will perform your One-Minute-in-the-Morning Energizer.
- ▶ Three times a week, you will do a 15- to 30-minute strength-training workout at home (or in a gym—your choice) using simple weights or exercise bands.
- ▶ **Optional exercise:** On days when you don't strength train, you may want to walk, run, bike, or do some other interval-style cardio exercise for 10 to 30 minutes.

Here's a Sample Schedule:

DAY 1
Full-body Tone and Strengthen workout (15 to 30 minutes)

DAY 2
Optional cardio interval workout (10 to 30 minutes)

DAY 3
Full-body Tone and Strengthen workout (15 to 30 minutes)

DAY 4
Optional cardio interval workout

DAY 5
Full-body Tone and Strengthen workout (15 to 30 minutes)

DAY 6
Optional cardio interval workout

DAY 7
Rest

EVERY DAY (even Day 7)
One-Minute-in-the-Morning Energizer

Don't panic: These workouts are short and simple, and so flexible that you can fit them in at any time of the day, and they'll work with whatever energy level and time constraints you're dealing with.

The One-Minute-in-the-Morning Energizer

If you are overweight and don't exercise regularly, the One-Minute-in-the-Morning Energizer is custom made for you. McMaster University researchers knew that intense brief bouts of hard exercise interspersed with much slower recovery segments provided a great metabolic lift to burn calories as well as improved measures of endurance and cardiovascular health. What they wanted to find out was the minimum effort you could exert to reap the fitness benefits of much longer exercise sessions. Thirty seconds of all-out effort is just too long for many overweight and out-of-shape people to manage so they tried cutting that intense segment by a third, and sure enough, it worked.

What this means for you: three 20-second bouts of all-out physical effort (or you might call it one cumulative minute of hell), in between slow, easy bouts of recovery movement, are all you need to gain significant physical benefits of exercise. It's quick and it will get you in the groove to move more during the day. Use your smartphone's stopwatch function or a second hand of a clock to keep track of your time. Here are a couple of ways to get it done:

On a stationary bike, treadmill, or other cardio machine:

2 minutes → warm up by pedaling or walking at an easy pace.

20 seconds → pedal, walk, or run as fast and hard as you can while maintaining control and good form.
We're talking about all-out effort. Don't hold anything back for a full 20 seconds. At the end, you should be huffing and puffing to catch your breath.

90 seconds → recovery movement. Slow way down to a very easy pace. Don't stop; keep pedaling or walking slowly until your breathing returns to a normal, comfortable rate.
As you near the 90-second mark, start to ramp up your intensity again.

20 seconds → high-intensity exercise.

90 seconds → recovery pace.

20 seconds → high-intensity exercise.

That's 6 minutes; you're done!

In a small room without exercise equipment:

2 minutes → warm up by marching in place. Swing your arms and lift your knees so your thighs rise to nearly parallel with the floor. Do this at an easy pace. It'll raise your heart rate a bit to warm up your muscles and joints.

20 seconds → intense exercise. Choose one of the following body weight exercises to do at a high level of effort.

90 seconds → recovery pace. March in place slowly until your breathing returns to normal.

20 seconds → intense exercise using the exercise of your choice.

90 seconds → recovery pace. March in place slowly until your breathing returns to normal.

20 seconds → intense exercise using the exercise of your choice.

You're finished!

Great Body-Weight Exercises for the 20-Second Intense Effort Interval (choose one):

Arms-Up Squat

- ▶ Spread your feet shoulder-width apart with toes pointed slightly outward. Raise both arms above your head.
- ▶ Keeping arms raised, bend your knees and push your butt back as if sitting in a chair.
- ▶ Lower your body until your thighs are parallel with the floor.
- ▶ Pause a second and quickly straighten your legs to stand.
- ▶ Repeat immediately and quickly for 20 seconds.

Superhero Squat Jump

- ▶ Do the arms-up squat as described above but from the squat position, explosively press your feet into the floor to jump as high as you can (or as high as your ceiling will allow).
- ▶ Repeat as fast as possible for 20 seconds.

SEAL Jack

These are the jumping jacks that Navy SEALS do, and they are great, especially for those who experience pain when raising arms overhead while doing traditional jumping jacks.

- ▶ Start by standing with your feet together and placing your palms on your chest with elbows spread and arms parallel with the floor.
- ▶ As you jump to spread your legs outward, simultaneously swing your arms out to the sides so they are parallel with the floor.
- ▶ Jump your feet back while swinging your arms back to your chest. Do these as quickly as you can for 20 seconds.

Push-up

This classic chest/arms/abs exercise will elevate your heart rate very quickly if done fast.

► Get into a plank position, with your arms straight, hands on the floor directly underneath your shoulders and your toes on the floor behind you. Your body should be arrow straight from your heels to your head.

► Without dipping or lifting your butt, lower yourself until your chest nearly touches the floor and then immediately press yourself back to the starting position and repeat for 20 seconds.

These are tough. To make them easier, you can do modified push-ups by either kneeling OR by placing your hands on the edge of a bathtub or chair, which will reduce the amount of weight you'll be pushing.

To make push-ups more metabolic, push off the floor explosively so that your hands come off the floor.

For an even greater challenge, throw in a clap before your hands return to the floor.

Reverse Lunge

► Stand straight with feet hip-width apart, hands on your hips. Take a big step backward with your right leg and press the ball of your right foot to the floor as you lower your body by bending your left leg.

► Lower until your left leg forms a right angle and your right knee hovers an inch above the floor.

► Next press back into a standing position and bring your right foot forward.

► Repeat the move by stepping back with your left foot. Continue alternating this way for 20 seconds.

To make this exercise more challenging, hold a lightweight dumbbell in each hand. Don't have weights? Hold a gallon jug of water in each hand as you do the exercise.

Mountain Climber

- ▶ Get into the "up" push-up position with your hands directly under your shoulders and arms straight.

- ▶ Now, rapidly bend and straighten each leg one at a time in alternating fashion. It's like running in place with your hands on the ground. Try bringing your knees to your chest with each pump of your legs.

- ▶ Do these as fast as possible for a full 20 seconds.

Burpee

This advanced exercise is similar to the squat thrusts you performed in high school gym class. And it's a great way to crank up the intensity.

- ▶ Stand with feet hip-width apart. Bend at the knees and waist to place your hands shoulder-width apart on the floor in front of you.

- ▶ Quickly jump your feet back so you end up in a plank position. (Optional step: Do a push-up at this point.)

- ▶ Then jump your feet back under you and straighten your legs to jump back to a standing position.

- ▶ Repeat rapidly for 20 seconds.

Do the energizer every morning and even on weekends. If you are very out of shape, this simple 6-minute session (1 minute hard/ 5 minutes easy) will help you build up your cardiovascular fitness very quickly. And you'll find a funny thing happening: You'll like the feeling and want to do more.

Tone and Strengthen Workout

Strength training builds stronger muscles. The type of strength training workout here will not give you the hulky bulky muscles that make you look like a comic-book superhero. By building stronger muscle mass in this plan, you will make your body look firmer, tighter, more toned, and healthier. Just what you want! And because muscle mass burns more calories than fat (not a lot, but every little bit counts!), the more muscle on your skeleton, the quicker you will lose the fat throughout your body, especially abdominal fat.

Strength training is doubly important as we age. With each passing decade, your body naturally loses muscle mass and, if you're not careful about reducing your calorie consumption accordingly, replaces it with fat.

Strength training and strong muscles offer many other health and weight-loss benefits:

► They boost your energy level, making everyday tasks easier.

► Strong muscles help your body react more quickly in emergency situations, like when you trip over a curb and need to step quickly to catch your balance before you do a face-plant on the sidewalk.

► Strength training triggers your body to grow stronger, denser bones, to combat the bone loss that accelerates especially in women as they age.

► Muscle helps your body metabolize blood sugar, reducing your risk of developing type 2 diabetes.

► Strength training improves sleep quality.

Are you convinced that strength training is something you absolutely must do not only to lose your belly rapidly but also to bulletproof your body as you get older? I am. That's why I developed this easy resistance workout that you can do at home or at the gym, especially for people who may not be familiar with traditional weight-training exercises.

This is a resistance workout, meaning you will stress your muscles against resistance caused by holding light dumbbells or jugs of water or using exercise bands. Stressing a muscle against resistance causes tiny pain-free microtears in muscle tissue. At night while you're asleep, your body will repair those microscopic injuries in a process that builds and strengthens muscle.

To do this workout at home, you'll need to purchase dumbbells and elastic fitness bands online or at a sporting-goods store. Dumbbells come in many different weights. A pair of 8- to 10-pound dumbbells will be fine for these exercises. Dumbbells hold one distinct advantage over their cousin the barbell. Because your hands aren't fixed in relation to each other, as with a barbell, dumbbells give the advantage of being able to work each side of your body independently of the other. The freedom of motion they allow helps you to work around any joint injuries or flexibility issues you may have. Plus, dumbbells help develop both symmetry and stability.

The exercise descriptions below are for dumbbells or filled plastic water jugs. You can easily adapt them if you are using resistance bands.

How to Do the Tone and Strengthen Workout

For a simple total-body strength workout, always begin with a 3-minute warm-up of either stationary cycling or body-weight calisthenics such as jumping jacks and skater hops. Next, do 3 sets of 8 to 12 repetitions of each of the following exercises. Rest for about 30 seconds between exercises. Complete each set of the same exercise before moving on to the next exercise.

Warm-Up

Jumping Jacks AND Skater Hops

Jumping Jacks

- ► Stand straight with your feet hip-width apart and hands at your sides.

- ► Simultaneously raise your arms above your head as you jump and spread your feet shoulder-width apart.

- ► Jump your feet back to center while lowering arms to your sides. Repeat quickly.

Skater Hops

- ► Start with feet together. Push off with your left foot to hop laterally to the right about 3 feet. Land on your right foot and follow by swinging your left behind you.

- ► Immediately hop back, pushing off your right foot, landing on your left and trailing your right behind you. Swing your arms with each hop in an ice-skating motion.

Strength Workout

Plank OR Push-up → 1 set for plank | 3 sets, 8–10 reps for push-up

Plank

- ▶ Get on all fours and then extend your legs out straight behind you. Your hands should be directly under your shoulders. Straighten your arms.

- ▶ Brace your core and keep your back flat, forming a straight line from your heels to your head.

- ▶ Hold this rigid position for 30 to 60 seconds.

Push-up

- ▶ Get into a plank position with your palms on the floor directly under your shoulders and your arms straight. Your back should be flat and rigid from your heels to your head.

- ▶ Brace your core. This will help you maintain proper form and burn more calories because you are engaging more muscle fibers.

- ▶ Bend your arms to lower yourself toward the floor until your chest is about an inch from the floor. Press yourself up explosively. Repeat.

- **Easier Alternative STEP PUSH-UP:** Get into a push-up position, but instead of placing your hands on the floor, place them on a stair step, bench, or other stable structure that's raised off the floor.

- ▶ Keep your back arrow straight from heels to head. Your arms should be extended straight. Brace your abs.

- ▶ Bend your elbows to lower yourself until your chest is an inch off the step. Pause a second, then push yourself up. Repeat.

Dumbbell Squat → 8–10 reps | 3 sets

► Hold a 10-pound dumbbell in each hand at your sides. Stand with your feet spread shoulder-width apart with toes pointed slightly outward.

► Bend your knees and push your butt back as if trying to close a door behind you. Lower your body until your thighs are parallel with the floor.

► Pause a second and quickly straighten your legs to stand. Repeat.

Flutter Kick → 10 reps | 3 sets

► Lie on your back on the floor with your arms palms-down next to your sides and your toes pointed.

► Engage your abs to lift your feet about a foot off the floor.

► Keeping your legs rigid, begin quickly flutter kicking your straight legs back and forth as you would while swimming. Every four kicks equals one rep. Do 10.

Dumbbell Biceps Curl → 8–10 reps | 3 sets

► Stand with feet hip-width apart and hold a 5- to 10-pound dumbbell in each hand at your sides, palms facing in.

► Simultaneously bend both arms to raise the dumbbells to your shoulders.

► As you slowly raise the weights, rotate your hands outward so your thumbs face away from your body by the time the weights reach the front of your shoulders.

Note: Your upper arms should remain stationary against your body throughout the movement.

► Pause, then slowly lower the weights, while rotating your hands inward so that your palms face toward the sides of your thighs by the time your arms are straight. Repeat.

Dumbbell Forward Lunge → 8-10 reps | 3 sets

▶ Stand with your feet together and hold a dumbbell in each hand at your sides, palms facing in.

▶ Take a large step forward with your right leg and lower your body toward the floor.

▶ Your front leg should bend at the knee, forming a right angle. Your back leg should be bent slightly. Lower yourself until you back knee hovers an inch above the ground and your right thigh is parallel with the floor. Pause in this position for a second.

▶ Press your right foot into the floor to push yourself back to the starting position.

▶ Next, step forward with your left foot and repeat.

Dumbbell Push Press → 8-10 reps | 3 sets

▶ Stand with your feet shoulder-width apart and hold a dumbbell in each hand at your shoulders, elbows bent, palms facing in.

▶ Bend your knees to dip down slightly into a half squat.

▶ Press your feet into the floor to aggressively stand while straightening your arms overhead. (Straightening your legs will provide momentum to help you press the weights overhead.)

▶ Slowly lower the weights to your shoulders and repeat.

Side Plank → (right side) 30- to 60-second hold | 1 set

▶ Lie on the floor on your right side, stack your left leg on top of your right, and prop yourself up on your right elbow and forearm. Your elbow should be directly under your shoulder. Place your left hand on your hip.

▶ Brace your core and lift your hips off the floor so that your body forms a rigid straight line. Don't allow your hips to sag. Hold this position for 30 to 60 seconds, then release to the floor.

Dumbbell Standing Triceps Press → 8–10 reps | 3 sets

▶ Stand with feet shoulder-width apart and hold a dumbbell in each hand.

▶ Press the dumbbells above your head so your arms are straight and your palms are facing in.

▶ Keeping your upper arms against your ears, move only your forearms by bending at the elbows to lower the weight simultaneously behind your head.

▶ Once your forearms meet your biceps, press the weights back until your arms are straight again, being careful to move only your forearms. Repeat.

Side Plank → (left side) 30- to 60-second hold | 1 set

▶ Lie on the floor on your left side, stack your right leg on top of your left, and prop yourself up on your left elbow and forearm. Your elbow should be directly under your shoulder. Place your right hand on your hip.

▶ Brace your core and lift your hips off the floor so that your body forms a rigid straight line. Don't allow your hips to sag. Hold this position for 30 to 60 seconds, then release to the floor.

YOUR MUSCLES ARE TALKING ABOUT YOU

In 2008, researchers first identified compounds called myokines, which are hormones produced by skeletal muscle that's secreted into the bloodstream in response to muscle contractions.

Myokines can do amazing things. Some help increase fat-burning in both the liver and skin tissue; others improve the function of the vascular system. Some improve the immune response; still others help our digestive system by improving communication between the pancreas and intestines. There's even some evidence that myokines released through exercise may influence cancer cell growth.

The mightiest source of myokines? You're sitting on it. The muscles of the legs and butt contract when we're upright. To accomplish that trick, they use stored sugar to fuel them-selves, simultaneously stimulating the release of compounds that improve our cholesterol levels and metabolism. The more time you spend on your feet, the more time you spend with these muscles contracted—and hence, the more time you spend shooting out myokines.

But which muscles make the most sense to focus on? The answer is in your butt: Our legs and backside contain some of the largest muscles in our body. As a result, they store—and burn—the most glycogen. An exercise routine that brings these large muscles into play will burn off larger amounts of glycogen, and cause a greater reduction in fat stores, than a routine in which you're working your arms or chest, for example.

Optional Cardio Workouts

Here's another great way to boost your fat-burning metabolism and improve your health without sacrificing muscle. This optional cardio workout uses the same high-intensity interval-training concept you employ with your One-Minute-in-the-Morning Energizer session. You alternate short bursts of faster, high-intensity activity with bouts of slower, less-intensity "recovery" periods.

Many studies have shown that this type of exercise is highly effective for weight loss and targeting belly fat. For example, consider this Danish study reported by the American Diabetes Association: Two groups of people with type 2 diabetes were put on a walking program; one group walked at a steady speed while the other group varied their walking speed. After four months, the interval-training group lost eight more pounds than the steady walkers. Even better, the walkers who changed up their speeds lost visceral belly fat and improved their blood sugar control.

Here's a simple speed walking interval that you can do in 10 minutes.

2 MINUTES → warm-up of slow, easy walking

30 SECONDS → **Walk fast,** pumping your arms to engage your entire body.

60 SECONDS → **Slow down to a moderate pace** to lower your heart rate.

60 SECONDS → **Walk fast.**

2 MINUTES → **Slow to a moderate pace.** You should be able to talk in complete sentences.

30 SECONDS → **Walk fast.**

3 MINUTES → **Slow to a moderate pace.**

30-Minute Walking Interval

3 MINUTES → warm-up of slow, easy effort

60 SECONDS → fast walk

2 MINUTES → slow, easy effort

60 SECONDS → fast walk

2 MINUTES → slow, easy effort

60 SECONDS → fast walk

2 MINUTES → slow, easy effort

60 SECONDS → fast walk

2 MINUTES → slow, easy effort

60 SECONDS → fast walk

2 MINUTES → slow, easy effort

60 SECONDS → fast walk

2 MINUTES → slow, easy effort

60 SECONDS → fast walk

2 MINUTES → slow, easy effort

60 SECONDS → fast walk

2 MINUTES → slow, easy effort

60 SECONDS → fast walk

60 SECONDS → slow, easy effort

60 SECONDS → fast walk

3 MINUTES → slow cooldown

10-Minute Stair-Climbing Interval

Another way to increase the metabolic intensity of a walking workout and shorten workout time is to make walking harder. Do that with a stair-climbing interval workout. Use the stadium bleachers of a local athletic field or your workplace stairs. You don't go very fast. Climbing the stairs will force your high-intensity effort. Staircases have roughly a 65 percent grade, which will force you to exert much more leg strength to lift your body weight.

► Warm up by walking on flat ground at a slow pace for 2 minutes.

► Walk up the stairs (at least ten stairs) quickly but in control.

► Walk down at a moderate pace and repeat.

To progress, try taking every other stair step going up. It's an explosive movement that generates a lot of leg power.

chapter

13

THE ZERO SUGAR WAY OF LIFE

How to Stay Lean Forever!

A SUCCESSFUL LIFE IS A MATTER OF HARNESSING MOMENTUM.

It's hard to start moving, as anyone who's ever said "Just let me lie down on the couch for a minute" can attest. It takes physical, mental, and emotional energy to alter one's speed and direction; in fact, a 2015 study found that more than half of the calorie burn that comes from a long walk actually comes from the stopping and starting you do, not from the stretches of walking in between.

People who build momentum and keep it moving in the right direction tend to succeed at things, and they tend to keep succeeding at them. People who fail to seize the day and fail to follow through invariably repeat that pattern time and time again—not because they're any less motivated, disciplined, or well-meaning, but because they've been sidetracked. Eat healthy and go to the gym today, and it will be much easier to do the same tomorrow. Give yourself over to a bon-bon festival on your couch, and you've already begun a pattern that will take considerable effort to break.

Isaac Newton—the guy who supposedly discovered gravity when an apple fell from a tree and bonked him on the head—created the Three Laws of Motion, which boil down to this: an object at rest tends to stay at rest, while an object in motion tends to stay in motion. That's true of meteors, and it's true of people, as well.

Fortunately, if you've made it this far through *Zero Sugar Diet*, you're already moving in the right direction, and you're probably carrying some serious momentum. Simply by following the Sustain program, you'll be able to continue your weight loss without having to carefully watch what you eat or give up most of your favorite foods.

But even the simplest and most effective plans can come unhinged if you allow yourself to break the pattern. We are creatures of habits, and those habits will either help us stay lean or cause us to gain weight.

So to help you continue building on your momentum, I've studied some of the recent and most compelling research on what makes people successful in keeping weight off, and boiled them down into a series of strategies that can help you continue to build on your success. For each one of these statements you can agree with, your chances of continuing your weight-loss journey only improve.

You don't cheat. "Cheat meals" are a common gimmick that a lot of diet plans use to help people deal with the challenges of sticking to a strict diet program. But cheat meals not only break your weight-loss momentum, they can also damage your health. In a study in *The FASEB Journal* in 2015, researchers took blood samples from volunteers who were struggling with obesity and those who were lean and healthy. Of course, the samples showed different readings in terms of cholesterol and blood sugar. Then, both groups were given a high-calorie shake. When blood was taken from them after the shake, those whose readings had been healthy earlier showed the same sort of elevated risk factors for heart disease and diabetes as the unhealthy group.

But you make sure to eat breakfast. In a 2011 national survey from the Calorie Control Council, 17 percent of Americans admitted to skipping meals to lose weight. The problem is, skipping meals actually increases your odds of obesity, especially when it comes to breakfast. A study from the *American Journal of Epidemiology* found that people who cut out the morning meal were 4.5 times more likely to be obese. Why? Skipping meals slows your metabolism and boosts your hunger. That puts your body in prime fat-storage mode and increases your odds of overeating at the next meal.

You eat dessert with a fork instead of a spoon. A 2016 study at the University of South Florida found that when people ate a chocolate cake with a spoon, they ate more of it and underestimated the number of calories they were consuming; when they used a fork, they consumed less and were better able to guess how much they'd eaten.

You sleep through the night. According to Wake Forest researchers, dieters who sleep five hours or less put on two and a half times more belly fat, while those who sleep more than eight hours pack on only slightly less than that. Shoot for an average of six to seven hours of sleep per night—the optimal amount for weight control. And while we've long known that missing a few hours of sleep can lead to weight gain, new science shows that the worst hours to miss are the ones that fall in the middle of the night. A recent study at Johns Hopkins University monitored the moods of people who dealt with different kinds of sleep deprivation. They found that those who simply got too little sleep had a 12 percent decrease in positive mood; those whose sleep was interrupted in the middle of the night suffered nearly three times as great an impact. The reason is that slow-wave sleep, the period needed for bodily repair, happens during the middle of your sleep cycle.

You prefer almond butter to peanut butter. Almonds may be the single best dietary source of vitamin E, and E might as well stand for "extra-slim." But as much as 92 percent of the American population doesn't get enough. Worse, people struggling with obesity actually have a harder time absorbing E than lean people do, according to a 2015 study in *The American Journal of Clinical Nutrition*. A spoonful of almond butter gives you three times as much vitamin E as the same amount of peanut butter.

You leave notes for yourself. Subtle, even subliminal, messages may be more effective at helping us stick to a healthy eating regimen than even ongoing, conscious focus, found a 2015 study in the *Journal of Marketing Research*. The study found that people who receive reinforcing notes urging them to eat healthily were more likely to make smarter choices than those who tried to keep their goals top of mind at all times. Simple reminders—keeping a bowl of nuts on your kitchen counter, for example, or putting reminders into your phone—will keep you on the winning side while your mind is busy tackling other things.

You wave off the bread. Breadsticks, biscuits, and chips and salsa may be complimentary at some restaurants, but that doesn't mean you won't pay for them. Every time you eat one of Olive Garden's free breadsticks or Red Lobster's Cheddar Bay Biscuits, you're adding an additional 150 calories to your meal. Eat three over the course of dinner and that's 450 calories. That's also roughly the number of calories you can expect for every basket of tortilla chips you get at your local Mexican restaurant. What's worse, none of these calories comes paired with any redeeming nutritional value. Consider them junk food on steroids.

You put your fork down between bites. If your body has one major flaw, this is it: It takes twenty minutes for your stomach to tell your brain that it's had enough. A study in the *Journal of the American Dietetic Association* found that slow eaters took in 66 fewer calories per meal, but compared to their fast-eating peers, they felt like they had eaten more. What's 66 calories, you ask? If you can do that at every meal, you'll lose more than twenty pounds a year! A simple trick to slow your pace: Simply place your fork down on the plate after each bite.

You only watch the tube when there's something special on. A University of Vermont study found that overweight participants who reduced their TV time by just 50 percent burned an additional 119 calories a day on average. That's an automatic twelve-pound annual loss! Maximize those results by multitasking while you watch—even light household tasks will further bump up your caloric burn. Plus, if your hands are occupied with dishes or laundry, you'll be less likely to mindlessly snack—the other main occupational hazard associated with tube time.

You make all your own food decisions. A study in the *Journal of Public Policy & Marketing* shows that compared to ordering à la carte, you pick up a hundred or more extra calories by opting for the "combo" or "value meal." Why? Because when you order items bundled together, you're likely to buy more food than you want. You're better off ordering your food piecemeal. That way, you won't be influenced by pricing schemes designed to hustle a few more cents out of your pocket.

At restaurants, you focus on the scenery. Cornell researchers found that when eating at a buffet-style restaurant, obese diners were 15 percent more likely to choose seats with a clear view of the food. Your move: Choose a seat that places your back toward the spread. It will help you avoid fixating on the food and turn your attention to people-watching.

You hassle your doctor. Although you may get scanned for high cholesterol or diabetes at your annual exam, MDs don't typically test or look for physical signs of nutritional deficiencies. Michelle Loy, MPH, MS, CSSD, Registered Dietitian Nutritionist, and owner of Go Wellness in Orange County, California, suggests having your vitamin

D levels checked if nothing else. "Many people are deficient and don't even know it—and not getting enough may increase the risk of osteoporosis, heart disease and certain types of cancer," she warns. Vitamin D has also been shown to improve exercise performance.

You look down. At the bathroom scale, that is. Looking at your body weight frequently reinforces weight-loss goals and makes it more difficult to cheat on your diet. When University of Minnesota researchers observed dieters who weighed themselves daily, they discovered that the routine of stepping on a scale helped those people lose twice as much weight as those who weighed themselves less frequently. Avoid being thrown off by natural fluctuations in body weight by stepping onto the scale the same time every day.

You keep ice water at your side at all times. In one University of Utah study, dieting participants who were instructed to drink two cups of water before each meal lost 30 percent more weight than their thirsty peers. Part of the reason: If you're not drinking ample water, your body may *have* to store carbs as fat. Your body cannot efficiently change carbs into energy without ample water. To boost the calorie-burning effects of H_2O, add ice. German researchers found that six cups of cold water a day could prompt a metabolic boost that incinerates 50 additional daily calories.

You order first at restaurants. If you want to take charge of your weight, take charge of your restaurant order. A University of Illinois study found that groups of people tend to order similarly, especially when forced to say their order out loud. That's one reason why research from *The New England Journal of Medicine* indicates that when a friend becomes obese, it ups your chance of obesity by 57 percent.

You have a stress outlet that's not food. A study from the University of Alabama found that emotional eaters—those who admitted eating in response to emotional stress—were thirteen times more likely to be overweight or obese. If you feel the urge to eat in response to stress, try chewing a piece of gum, chugging a glass of water, or taking a walk around the block. Create an automatic response that doesn't involve food and you'll prevent yourself from overloading on calories.

You mix up your carbs. Modern diet gurus have made carbs seem so scary, it's no wonder the health-conscious among us are afraid to venture too far from the quinoa. But new research shows that your fat-burning system actually operates better when you keep it guessing, so don't let yourself get caught in a rut. Eating a variety of carbs is actually desirable, at least for athletes, according to the journal *Essentials of Strength Training and Conditioning*. Keep in mind, that's not an invitation to gorge on Froot Loops. Instead, try focusing more on "wet" carbs, especially at night. What's a "wet" carb? That means carbs that have high amounts of water in them, such as cucumbers, leafy green salads, tomatoes, and steamed asparagus. Wet carbs allow you to maintain relatively adequate levels of water during the night since you can't drink while you sleep. Staying hydrated overnight means your body will continue to get the nourishment it needs to unveil your abs even while you're dreaming of a faraway beach.

You get to work early and leave on time. When deadlines pile up, add work hours to the beginning of your day, not the end. When you work later you also eat later and go to sleep later, both of which lead to unwanted pounds. A study in the journal *Nutrition Research* found that those whose last meal was closest to bedtime took in more calories overall throughout the day than those who gave their bodies time to recover before heading off to bed.

You never drive to work. Those who drive to work gain more weight than those who take public transportation, according to a study in the *British Medical Journal*. According to the study, commuting by car slaps an extra 5.5 pounds on your body, whether you exercise or not. Ouch. Another study in Japan found that people who take public transportation to work were 44 percent less likely to be overweight, 27 percent less likely to have high blood pressure, and 34 percent less likely to have diabetes.

You walk the halls. We sit an average of sixty-seven hours a week—

that's nine hours a day sitting, eight hours lying down, and only about seven hours out of every twenty-four spent actually moving. And our sedentary jobs now cause us to burn 100 fewer calories a day than we did fifty years ago. That alone translates to gaining an extra ten pounds a year. But a recent study in the *Clinical Journal of the American Society of Nephrology* found that taking a two-minute walk every hour can offset the effects of too much sitting. Make it a habit to never call a colleague when you can just as easily stop by his or her office to talk.

You get outside every morning. In studies, sun exposure between 8:00 a.m. and noon is associated with higher fat burning and significantly lower BMIs, regardless of exercise, calorie intake, sleep, or even age. If mornings are hectic, at least open the blinds in the a.m., especially at work. Employees with windows near their desks receive 173 percent more white light exposure during work hours and forty-six more minutes of sleep per night than employees who don't have exposure to natural light. And those without windows get less physical activity. Plus, a new study in *Proceedings of the National Academy of Sciences* found that being exposed to artificial light leads to weight gain regardless of what you eat.

You decompress between work and home. A recent study in the *American Journal of Epidemiology* found that people with high levels of job stress are 26 percent more likely to be inactive during their downtime than those with low-stress jobs. A University of Rochester study echoed these results, finding that stress at work leads to unhealthy behaviors like more sitting and watching TV and less exercise. If tension runs high at your office, create an active barrier that keeps you from dropping right onto the couch when you get home.

You eat grapefruit. While the exact mechanism is unclear, grapefruit seems to have a particularly powerful effect on weight loss. A study printed in the journal *Metabolism* found that eating half a grapefruit before meals may help reduce visceral fat and lower cholesterol levels. Participants in the six-week study who ate a Rio Red grapefruit fifteen minutes before breakfast, lunch, and dinner saw their waists shrink by up to an inch, and LDL levels drop by 18 points. Researchers attribute the effects to a combination of phytochemicals and vitamin C in the grapefruit. Consider having half of one before your morning oatmeal, slicing a few segments for a starter salad, or eat one for a snack shortly before a meal.

You wear jeans to work. A study by the American Council on Exercise suggests that casual clothing, as opposed to conventional business attire, can increase physical activity levels in our daily routines. Participants in the study took an additional 491 steps and burned 25 more calories, on days they wore denim than when wearing traditional suit wear. That may sound trivial, but the calories add up! Researchers say keeping it casual just once a week could slash 6,250 calories over the course of the year—enough to offset the average annual weight gain (0.4 to 1.8 pounds) experienced by most Americans.

You snack after, not before, lunch. A study published in the *Journal of the American Dietetic Association* found that mid-morning snackers tended to consume more throughout the day than afternoon snackers. Afternoon snackers, on the other hand, tend to choose good snacks.

chapter 14

THE ZERO SUGAR 3-DAY DETOX

How to Turbocharge Your Results in Just One Weekend!

FIRST, BEFORE WE START THIS CHAPTER about my detox cleanse, a word about detox cleanses:

They're a hoax.

Okay, there, I said it. Whether it's the Master Cleanse or the Grapefruit Diet or any plan that has you living for a week on nothing but green smoothies or baby food, no fast or cleanse will do anything in particular to "detoxify" your body. And worse, some may even wind up depriving your body of critical nutrients, in particular calcium and fiber.

For example, consider juice fasts, in which you give up solid food and live on juiced fruits and vegetables—using protocols that are often built around a balance of different kinds of juices designed to battle inflammation, ease digestion, and boost immunity. Juice Press, for example, will sell you a five-day cleanse for just $360 (including "cleanse waters"). The company claims the cleanse will reduce cell damage, relieve stress on your heart, and lead to "better well-being," among other things. All you have to do is give up solid food and live exclusively on their juice.

Now, there are definite upsides to any plan that boosts your intake of leafy greens and other fruits and vegetables while reducing the amount of saturated fat, preservatives, and sodium you take in. But juicing isn't the way to do it. You've just read an entire book about the value of fiber and how it can help immunize your body from the damaging effects of sugar. So does it make sense to do a "cleanse" involving just juice, in which all of the fiber has been stripped away—leaving nothing but the sugar behind?

Additionally, there's never been a conclusive study showing that dietary cleanses actually "cleanse" anything: One small German study way back in 2003 found that after an eight-day juice cleanse, subjects had some moderate improvement in blood cholesterol; a week later, however, their levels had returned to normal.

The fact is, your body is an amazing instrument, one with an entire series of organs—the excretory system—dedicated to doing nothing but detoxifying the whole works, 24/7. No matter how much nutritional abuse you want to heap on yourself, your body will continue slaving away, liver and kidneys working overtime to get rid of the junk you throw their way. And despite what you may have heard, there are no mysterious toxins or leftover bits of Big Macs lingering in the dark recesses of your body that three days of drinking juice or eating nothing but cabbage soup will clean out.

What a "Detox Cleanse" Really Does

Yet if you have friends who do detox cleanses, or if you've tried them yourself, you may strongly disagree with everything I've just said. In fact, a lot of people report not just accelerated weight loss but also higher energy levels, a greater sense of focus, and even a reduction in skin problems and allergies after performing a cleanse. What gives?

In reality, there's no magic elixir in juice, or in any other cleanse; nor is your body being "flushed of toxins" in any way. But a cleanse does one thing right: It eliminates most of the additives, preservatives, sodium, trans fats, added sugars, and other nasty things that have settled onto our food supply and mucked it up like seagulls at a beach picnic. A sensible cleanse combines healthy, natural foods and liquids and ensures you're getting a complete balance of nutrients. By dramatically restricting both the amount and the kinds of foods you eat, a healthy cleanse will:

▶ Reduce bloating and water retention because of its low sodium levels and high water volume.

▶ Reduce inflammation by eliminating unhealthy oils, added sugars, artificial preservatives, and other refined and man-made food products that have been linked to inflammatory responses.

▶ Improve your energy levels by reducing the ups and downs of insulin response—again, by limiting sugar and overall calorie intake.

▶ Speed weight loss through a combination of reduced inflammation, reduced calories, and reduced water retention.

▶ Clear up your skin, your stuffiness, your headaches, and any other nagging feelings by cutting gluten, dairy, artificial colors, and other foods that might be triggering allergies or food sensitivities you're not even aware of.

In other words, it's not your body that's being cleansed or detoxed—it's your food. And if the foods and drinks you consume during the cleanse also bolster your nutritional intake, all the better. I just want to make sure you understand that there's nothing magic about the food you're eating on any given cleanse, and nothing filthy or demonic hanging out inside of you that needs an exorcism.

So, are you ready for a healthy, three-day dose of reality?

Why the Three-Day Zero Sugar Detox Cleanse?

If you're anything like me, you tend toward impatience. Fortunately, when it comes to weight loss, impatience is a virtue.

Earlier, I outlined the reasons why losing weight quickly made

DON'T DETOX YOUR BODY—DETOX YOUR KITCHEN!

While your body does a fine job cutting the clutter from your interior, the same can't necessarily be said for how you manage your exterior, in particular your living space. And recent research has found that when you're surrounded by chaos, you're more likely to create chaos inside as well.

In early 2016, researchers divided a set of ninety-eight women into two groups. Both groups were asked to wait for another person in a kitchen, which was stocked with bowls of cookies, crackers, and carrots.

The difference is that one half of the women were waiting in a messy kitchen, one with piles of dirty dishes and papers scattered around. Researchers even made the phone ring in order to up the level of chaos. The other half of the women waited in the same kitchen with the same snacks, but the room had been neatened up, with all the dishes and clutter put away.

After ten minutes of waiting, the women who were trapped in the chaotic environment downed an additional 53 calories from cookies—twice as many cookies as the women in the neat and calm kitchen.

sense; studies show repeatedly that fast results are linked to lasting, long-term success. So I'm all in favor of doing a "cleanse" to jump-start your weight loss and help you take control of your health and your diet.

But the trick with any cleanse is to make sure that it's just the beginning of a healthy eating strategy that you can continue for the long run. In fact, in a 2016 study in the journal *Advances in Nutrition*, researchers at the University of California, Los Angeles, looked at twenty people who followed a three-day juice fast and found that there was a "significant decrease in weight and body mass index (BMI)" at day four. Huzzah!

The catch: Once the cleanse ended, the subjects went back to their normal way of eating. And, not unexpectedly, by day fourteen the subjects were back to their normal weight as well.

So consider the detox cleanse outlined in this chapter as a valuable weapon to fall back on any time you need to drop a few pounds quickly, whether it's for an upcoming pool party, a glamorous wedding, or any event at which you might run into a scheming ex who needs to get a good look at what he or she gave up.

Principles of the Three-Day Detox Cleanse

This cleanse is, at its heart, no different from the overall program outlined in this book, with one exception: It lasts only three days instead of fourteen.

And it won't be that hard. In fact, by eliminating added sugars completely, you may find that you emerge from this long weekend with your sweet tooth broken for good. For certain, you'll find that the standard, sugary fare you're used to eating will be almost achingly sweet, and you may naturally begin to adjust your diet to eliminate added sugars for good. Here's what you need to keep in mind:

► **Remember your big three:** Each meal and snack will still contain the three key elements of *Zero Sugar Diet*:

> A Power Protein
>
> A Flat-Belly Fat
>
> A source of fiber

► **Eliminate convenience foods:** There will be no prepackaged meals or snacks allowed; everything on this plan is convenient, but it's also a whole food, unadulterated by additives, preservatives, or, most important of all, sugars. If you need to swap something in or out, make sure you're substituting something with only one ingredient. If it's packaged fruit, make sure it's just fruit; if it's peanut butter, make sure it's made from only peanuts.

► **Cook once, eat thrice:** To help keep fiber and protein high, and calories low, I've used quinoa in each of the lunches over these three days. To make your life simple, just cook up a batch before starting the cleanse, and store it in the fridge, adding it into the recipes as directed.

► **Drink, drink, drink!** Throughout this cleanse, it's important to stay hydrated, so be sure to drink a glass of water or two before each meal, and more water throughout the day. Water helps you to feel full, allowing you to make healthier food choices. Plus, a lot of what we perceive as hunger is often just thirst. A 2015 study in the journal *Obesity* compared two groups of obese people and gave them the same weight-loss guidelines, except for one difference: Half of the subjects were instructed to drink about 16 ounces of water before each meal. At the end of twelve weeks, the water drinkers had lost an average of three pounds more than those who weren't told to drink up.

THE THREE-DAY SUGAR-FREE CLEANSE

DAY 1

Breakfast

2 sunny-side-up eggs topped with

+ ½ small avocado, sliced

Lunch

Thai bowl:

½ cup cooked quinoa

+ ¼ cup shredded carrots

+ ¼ cup cubed cucumber

+ 3 oz cubed tofu

+ 1 Tbsp chopped cilantro

+ 2 Tbsp salted peanuts

+ lime juice

Snack

Small apple

+ 2 Tbsp almond butter

Dinner

½ cup chopped fennel sautéed in garlic and extra-virgin olive oil
with ½ cup grape tomatoes and 3 cups baby spinach topped with
4 oz grilled chicken breast and ¼ cup black olives

DAY 2

Breakfast

Green dream smoothie:

½ cup baby spinach

+ ½ small avocado

+ ¼ cup frozen pineapple

+ ¼ cup raw cashews

+ 1 cup unsweetened almond milk

Lunch

Veggie nicoise bowl:

½ cup cooked quinoa

+ 1 hard-boiled egg, chopped

+ ¼ cup white cannellini beans

+ 8 green beans, chopped

+ ¼ cup chopped cherry tomato

+ 5 black olives

+ 2 tsp extra-virgin olive oil

+ 1 tsp red wine vinegar

Snack

¼ cup raw almonds

+ 1 small orange

Dinner

3 oz grilled wild salmon

+ 2 small sprouted corn tortillas

+ ½ cup shredded red cabbage

+ ¼ of a mango, chopped

+ lime juice

DAY 3

Breakfast

Savory oatmeal:

Prepare ½ cup dry rolled oats with water and a pinch of salt.
Mix in ¼ cup frozen peas and cook for 1 minute more.
Top with ¾ cup sautéed mushrooms.

Lunch

California bowl:

½ cup cooked quinoa

+ 3 oz cooked turkey or chicken breast, chopped

+ ¼ cup chopped red bell pepper

+ ¼ avocado, sliced

+ 2 Tbsp sunflower seeds

Snack

1 pear

+ 2 Tbsp cashew butter

Dinner

Escarole and white bean soup (makes 2 servings):

Sauté 1 medium head of escarole, chopped with garlic, extra-virgin
olive oil, and a pinch of dried red pepper flakes. Add a drained
and rinsed can of white cannellini beans and 2 cups of chicken or
vegetable broth. Simmer. Add salt and pepper to taste.

THE UNDIRTY DOZEN

The inside of your body is like the outside of your cat: It needs no help in cleaning itself, and, quite frankly, it doesn't take too well to your attempts to pitch in. A simple, healthy diet—one that's high in fiber and low in sugar, preservatives, and unhealthy fats—is all that's needed to keep your body's interior as smooth and sleek as the day it rolled off the assembly line.

But that doesn't mean the occasional boost isn't helpful, especially when you've been overindulging in your bad habits of choice. Here are twelve foods that can help your body recover from an excess of abuse.

ASPARAGUS

It's a natural diuretic, so asparagus can help relieve bloating and other unpleasant feelings. Its balance of amino acids and minerals may also help to alleviate hangover symptoms, according to a study in the *Journal of Food Science.*

AVOCADO

The superfruits contain two oils, linalool and geranyl acetate, that have been shown to have a positive effect on irritable bowel syndrome and other digestive disorders. In a study in the *Journal of Agricultural and Food Chemistry,* researchers fed twenty-two different fruits to a group of rats that had suffered liver damage. The avocado was the most beneficial in restoring liver function.

BANANAS

Thanks to their potent dose of potassium, bananas can help counterbalance the effects of sodium and reduce water retention. They're also packed with resistant starch, which helps to feed the healthy bacteria in your gut.

BEETS

These ruby-red roots contain a type of antioxidant called betalains that help repair and regenerate cells in the liver, your body's primary detox organ.

CITRUS PEEL

The skins of lemons, limes, and other citrus fruit contain an antioxidant d-limonene, which has been shown to help stimulate liver enzymes, according to the World Health Organization.

COLLARD GREENS

There might be a reason why collards are often served alongside fried chicken. Nutrients in the greens bind to bile acids in the body, helping to block the buildup of cholesterol in the bloodstream, according to a study in *Nutrition Research.*

DIJON MUSTARD

For a mere 5 calories, a teaspoon of mustard can boost metabolism by up to 25 percent for several hours, according to English researchers. Just make sure you're eating pure mustard, not the sweetened, honey mustard stuff!

GRAPEFRUIT

In one Japanese study, researchers found that grapefruit can enhance the action of calorie-burning brown fat cells, enhancing the breakdown of fat while reducing appetite. And a second study in the journal *Metabolism* found that eating half a grapefruit a day can whittle your middle by up to an inch in just six weeks.

KIWI

One of the few foods that combine fiber and omega-3 fatty acids, kiwi will help bolster your digestive system while reducing inflammation and improving heart health.

SARDINES

A three-week study in the *International Journal of Cardiology* found that smokers who supplemented with just 2 grams of omega-3s a day—about what you'd get in a 4-ounce serving of sardines—showed marked improvement in the elasticity of their arteries.

TURMERIC

The compound curcumin, found in the bright-orange Indian spice turmeric, has been shown to reduce bile duct blockage and scarring in the liver by interfering with chemical reactions involved in the inflammatory process, according to a study in the journal *Gut.*

WHITE TEA

A study in the journal *Nutrition & Metabolism* found that white tea can simultaneously stimulate the breakdown of fat in the body while blocking the formation of new fat cells.

chapter # 15

FREQUENTLY ASKED QUESTIONS

What's the difference between added sugars and natural sugars?

Sadly, sugar is sugar, no matter where it comes from—organic, raw, refined, etc. The sugar you consume naturally through whole fruits and vegetables will break down into the same molecules as the added sugars found in processed food. However, the sugars that occur naturally in the fruits and vegetables come with lots of benefits such as fiber, vitamins, and minerals, which slows the absorption of sugar into your bloodstream. Sugar from whole fruits and vegetables is always a better choice than added sugars, which provide zero nutrition benefits and extra calories.

How do I know if a food contains sugar?

Sugar may be obvious or it may be hidden. There are dozens of names you might find in the ingredients list that really just mean sugar. The USDA lists the following as alternate names for added sugars recognized by the FDA: anhydrous dextrose, brown sugar, confectioners' powdered sugar, corn syrup, corn syrup solids, dextrose, fructose, high-fructose corn syrup (HFCS), honey, invert sugar, lactose, malt syrup, maltose, maple syrup, molasses, nectars, pancake syrup, raw sugar, sucrose, sugar, white granulated sugar; other names not recognized by the FDA include: cane juice, evaporated corn sweetener, crystal dextrose, glucose, liquid fructose, sugar cane juice, and fruit nectar. Best bet: Use *Zero Sugar Diet*'s list of approved foods, in this book or at thezerosugardiet.com.

How do I know how much sugar is in a food?

You must read the Nutrition Label. Look at grams of sugar, then divide this by 4 to get that amount in teaspoons. For example, a can of cola may contain 40 grams of sugar. Dividing this by 4, we know that this can of soda has ten teaspoons of sugar. That is already over the recommended daily limit! You're best off choosing foods with ZERO added sugars.

I know this diet isn't about calorie counting per se, but how many calories does sugar have—I'm curious?

All carbohydrates have 4 calories in each gram. So that same can of cola that has 40 grams of sugar gives you 160 calories JUST FROM THE SUGAR! That is why we say "empty calories." There is absolutely nothing good that added sugar offers your body; it just gives us calories.

Even plain yogurt has sugar. Is it off the table?

No. Naturally occurring sugars in whole fruits and dairy products like milk and yogurt aren't an issue. We're looking at "added sugars," which means any kind of sugar that's listed on the ingredients, whether it's honey, sugar, molasses, agave, corn syrup, etc.

Can we have tea or coffee? Caffeine or no caffeine? Any natural sweeteners like organic honey or organic pure maple syrup?

Coffee and especially tea are powerful weight-loss drinks. You may consume as much as you like on this plan. Caffeinated or decaffeinated are fine. Natural sweeteners contain some form of sugar, and since there is no fiber in coffee or tea, using them would land your beverage in the Danger Zone. Please drink your coffee or tea without sweeteners. The plan allows for a limited amount of full-fat dairy products, so you may use milk. Alternatively, a squeeze of lemon in your tea can actually enhance its weight-loss powers.

How many grams of fiber am I getting per day? How many grams of sugar?

This fourteen-day plan will reduce added sugar down to no more than 10 percent of calories, or between 25 and 43 grams per day, maximum. The USDA recommends no more than 45 grams per day for women and 50 grams per day for men. On this plan, fiber is dependent on food choices but should be between 30 and 50 grams per day, depending on your sugar intake.

Can I eat "sugar-free" versions of foods?

No. "Sugar free" baked goods, candies, and the like are made with artificial sweeteners, which your brain interprets as sugar. As a result, it triggers a release of insulin that causes fat storage, just as if you'd eaten the sugar in the first place.

Most fruit has more sugar than fiber. Why is that okay on this plan?

It's only unnatural added sugars that we're concerned with. Two exceptions: fruit juices, because they have all the fiber stripped out of them, and dried fruits, because they are usually sweetened with added sugars.

I'm trying to be gluten-free. I found some gluten-free breads, but it seems like they have added sugar. Any suggestions on what to use for GF?

Gluten-free breads are acceptable, if you must, provided they meet the requirement of containing as much fiber as sugar. We like Food For Life gluten-free breads.

Do you want all of the foods to be organic?

Organic foods are great because they are grown without pesticides, which have been linked to weight gain in some cases. We recommend choosing them whenever possible. However, *Zero Sugar Diet* does not rely on your diet consisting only of organic foods.

I usually have a Shakeology shake for breakfast. I always use almond milk, then add fresh fruit and some flaxseed. May I still do that?

According to the nutrition information provided by the manufacturer, many Shakeology shakes contain more grams of sugar than they do fiber, making them inappropriate for the Zero Sugar Diet. In general, try to avoid packaged ingredients whenever possible; they often come with unnecessary chemicals and other additives. There are plenty of great, all-natural smoothie recipes in this book.

Appendix

THE NO-SUGAR AISLE-BY-AISLE SHOPPING GUIDE

WHEN I SET OUT TO WRITE *ZERO SUGAR DIET*, and suggested followers give up added sugar completely for fourteen days, my colleagues called me crazy: They thought I'd never be able to find enough name-brand supermarket foods that have no added sugar!

This section is devoted to them—and to you.

Using this list, researched exclusively for *Zero Sugar Diet*, you can feed your whole family delicious, nutritious foods, and easily eat no added sugars for fourteen days and beyond. Added bonus: You'll encourage the food manufactures to make more products like them.

So welcome to the ultimate sugar-free shopping list. We'll start where all grocery stores do: the produce aisle.

FRUITS

Although all fruits are allowed on *Zero Sugar Diet*, consider limiting yourself to two to three servings a day, since many are high in sugars, natural though they may be. For example, raspberries have only 5 grams of sugar per serving, while blackberries and strawberries have 7 grams—but apricots have 15 grams; grapefruit, pineapple, and kiwis have 16 grams; and bananas have 18 grams. Enjoy them, just don't eat twenty a day.

Apple	Fig	Papaya
Apricot	Goji Berry	Passion fruit
Avocado	Gooseberry	Peach
Banana	Grape	Pear
Blackberry	Grapefruit	Persimmon
Black currant	Guava	Pineapple
Blueberry	Honeydew	Pomegranate
Cantaloupe	Jackfruit	Pomelo
Cherimoya	Kiwi	Prune
Cherry	Kumquat	Quince
Cranberry	Lemon	Rambutan
Date	Lime	Raspberry
Dragon Fruit	Lychee	Star Fruit
Durian	Mango	Strawberry
Elderberry	Nectarine	Watermelon
	Orange	

VEGETABLES

As with fruits, all vegetables are Zero Sugar–friendly. But FYI, these have 5 grams of sugar or less, making them ideal: asparagus, bell pepper, broccoli, carrots, cauliflower, celery, cucumber, green beans, cabbage, leafy greens, mushrooms, potato, summer squash, corn, tomato.

Artichoke
Arugula
Bamboo Shoot
Beet Greens
Beets
Bell Pepper
Bitter Melon
Bok Choy
Broccoli
Broccoli Rabe
Broccolini
Brussels Sprouts
Cabbage
Capers
Carrot
Cauliflower
Celeriac
Celery
Chayote
Chicory
Chives
Collard Greens
Corn
Cucumber

Daikon
Dandelion Greens
Dill
Eggplant
Endive
Fiddlehead Ferns
Garlic
Garlic Chives
Ginger
Jerusalem Artichoke
Jicama
Kale
Kohlrabi
Lamb's Lettuce
Leek
Lettuce
Lotus Root
Olive
Parsnip
Pearl Onion
Peas
Potato
Pumpkin

Purslane
Radicchio
Radish
Rhubarb
Rutabaga
Salsify
Scallion
Shallot
Snap Pea
Snow Pea
Spinach
Squash
Squash Blossoms
Sweet Potato
Swiss Chard
Tatsoi
Tomato
Turnip
Water Chestnut
Watercress
Yam
Zucchini

POULTRY

Look for lean cuts with no additives.

Chicken
Duck
Goose
Ostrich

Pheasant
Quail
Turkey

MEATS

My favorite meats are grass-fed, pasture raised, minimally processed, and lean, and I like them fresh from the butcher counter or frozen without anything added.

Beef

Beerwurst

Bison

Bratwurst

Braunschweiger

Frog Legs

Game Meats

Ham

Lamb

Pate

Pepperoni

Pork

Veal

SEAFOOD

My seafood favorites are salmon (wild), trout (farmed), sardines (Pacific), anchovy, catfish (U.S.), herring (Atlantic), clams, shrimp, and mussels.

Anchovies

Carp

Catfish

Caviar

Cisco

Cod

Croaker

Eel

Flatfish

Haddock

Halibut

Herring

Jellyfish (dried, salted)

Mackerel

Mollusks

  Abalone

  Clam

  Conch

  Mussel

  Octopus

  Oyster

  Scallop

  Snail

  Squid

  Whelk

Mullet

Ocean Perch

Perch

Pike

Pollock

Pompano

Rockfish

Roe

Roughy, Orange

Salmon

Sardines

Scup

Seabass

Shad

Shark

Shellfish

  Crab

  Crayfish

  Lobster

  Shrimp

Smelt

Snapper

Sturgeon

Surimi

Swordfish

Trout

Tuna

Whitefish

Whiting

DAIRY

Butter & Margarine

Although it's sugar-free, I just can't recommend margarine, "light" butter, or anything with hydrogenated oils or trans fats. I prefer real butter (from grass-fed cows) or an olive oil/canola oil butter blend. The fewer the ingredients the better; real butter has only trace amounts of lactose.

Kerrygold
Land O' Lakes Butter with Canola Oil
Land O' Lakes Butter with Olive Oil
Organic Valley Cultured Butter
Smart Balance with Extra Virgin Olive Oil
Tin Star Foods Grass-Fed Brown Butter

Cheese

Most cheeses are naturally very low in sugar due to the fermentation process that produces it.

Milk

Since milk has naturally occurring sugar (lactose = glucose + galactose) and no added sugar, it can be enjoyed on *Zero Sugar Diet*, although it has 13 grams of sugar per cup.

Yogurt

If it's flavored—or in a flip cup—your yogurt is too high in sugar, so avoid all sweetened varieties (yes, even those sweetened with honey). Indulge instead in plain yogurt—especially Greek style—and top with delicious fresh fruits. "Sugar-free" yogurts contain artificial sweeteners that may be more harmful than regular sugar.

Brown Cow Greek Smooth and Creamy Plain
Chobani Plain
Fage Total 0%, 2%, or Whole Plain
Greek Gods Yogurt Nonfat Plain
Kanola Supernatural Plain
Maple Hill Creamery Greek Yogurt Plain

Oikos Traditional Plain
Oikos Triple Zero Greek Nonfat Yogurt
Siggi's 0% Plain
Wallaby Organic Purely Unsweetened Whole Milk Greek Yogurt

Eggs

One day, a mad scientist will find a way to inject sugar into an uncracked egg. Until that eggpocalypse, enjoy them freely.

Cereals

Give Honey Smacks the smackdown and tell the Cap'n to walk the plank—these cereals are hearty, satisfying, and sugar-free.

Arrowhead Mills Bulgur Wheat
Arrowhead Mills Oat Bran Hot Cereal
Arrowhead Mills Organic Gluten Free Rice and Shine Hot Cereal
Arrowhead Mills Puffed Barley
Arrowhead Mills Puffed Corn
Arrowhead Mills Puffed Kamut
Arrowhead Mills Puffed Millet
Arrowhead Mills Puffed Rice
Arrowhead Mills Steel Cut Oats Hot Cereal
Barbara's Shredded Wheat
Cream of Rice
Cream of Wheat Original
Cream of Wheat Whole Grain
Ezekiel 4:9 Sprouted Whole Grain Cereal Original
Ezekiel 4:9 Sprouted Whole Grain Cereal Golden Flax
General Mills Fiber One Original
Malt-O-Meal Creamy Hot Wheat
Malt-O-Meal Original Hot Wheat
Post Shredded Wheat Big Biscuit
Post Shredded Wheat 'n Bran
Post Shredded Wheat Original Spoon Size
Quaker Oats Old Fashioned
Quaker Puffed Rice
Quaker Puffed Wheat

BREADS

"Sugar free" doesn't mean you're free and clear: The second ingredient in a loaf of "sugar free" Nature's Own bread, for example, is maltitol, an artificial sweetener that leads to bloating. Search instead for sprouted breads, often found in your freezer aisle, like the ones below.

Ezekiel 4:9 Flax Sprouted Whole Grain Bread
Ezekiel 4:9 Whole Grain Bread
Joseph's Whole Wheat Pita Bread
Manna Organics Banana Walnut Hemp
Manna Organics Carrot Raisin
Manna Organics Cinnamon Date
Manna Organics Fig Fennel Flax
Manna Organics Fruit & Nut
Manna Organics Millet Rice
Manna Organics Multigrain
Manna Organics Sunseed Bread
Manna Organics Whole Rye

DELI MEATS

There's corn in your meat—in the form of dextrose, a sweetener. Slice sugar out of your diet with these, instead.

Applegate Natural Black Forest Ham
Applegate Natural Herb Turkey Breast
Applegate Natural Roast Beef
Applegate Natural Roasted Turkey Breast
Applegate Natural Smoked Turkey Breast
Applegate Organic Roasted Turkey Breast
Boar's Head All Natural Cap-Off Top Round Oven Roasted Beef
Boar's Head Beef Knockwurst (Natural Casing)
Boar's Head Beef Salami
Boar's Head Cocktail Beef Frankfurters (Natural Casing)
Boar's Head Deluxe Low Sodium Roasted Beef— Cap-Off Top Round
Boar's Head 1st Cut Cooked Corned Beef Brisket
Boar's Head Regular or Lite Beef Frankfurters (Natural Casing)
Boar's Head Regular or Lite Beef Frankfurters (Skinless)

HOT DOGS AND SAUSAGES

Oscar Mayer must think you're a wiener: They've loaded their dogs with two types of added sugars—corn syrup and dextrose! Go with these winners instead:

Hot Dogs

Applegate Natural Beef and Pork Hot Dog

Applegate Natural Big Apple Hot Dog

Applegate Natural Uncured Beef Hot Dog

Applegate Natural Uncured Chicken Hot Dog

Applegate Natural Uncured Turkey Hot Dog

Applegate The Great Organic Beef Hot Dog

Applegate The Great Organic Chicken Hot Dog

Applegate The Great Organic Stadium Beef Hot Dog

Applegate The Great Organic Turkey Hot Dog

Hebrew National Beef Franks

Pederson's No Sugar Uncured Beef Hotdogs

Sausages

Applegate Organics Sweet Italian

Pederson's Andouille Chicken Sausage

Pederson's No Sugar Chorizo Ground Sausage

Pederson's No Sugar Italian Ground Sausage

CONDIMENTS

Mayonnaise

Spectrum Organic Mayonnaise

Primal Kitchen Mayo with Avocado Oil

Ketchup

It's nearly impossible to find ketchup without some form of added sugar. It's part of the recipe. Even some homemade recipes call for honey or maple syrup.

Mustard

Annie's Organic Yellow Mustard
French's Deli Spicy Brown Mustard
Grey Poupon Dijon Mustard
OrganicVille Dijon Mustard No Added Sugar

Horseradish

Boar's Head Horseradish Grated in Vinegar

Vinegars

Try vinegars as condiments—wine vinegars, apple cider vinegar, and white vinegar add astringency and bite without the sugar.

GRAINS AND NOODLES

Rice

All rice is sugar-free—choose a whole grain while on *Zero Sugar Diet* and avoid white rice. Never buy boxed blends and mixes like Rice-A-Roni, which have added sugars such as maltodextrin.

Pasta

Twirl wisely: White pastas are nothing but refined carbs, which are no better than refined sugars. But any whole-grain pasta will do. Here are some of my favorite brands for Italian night.

Barilla ProteinPlus Angel Hair
Barilla ProteinPlus Spaghetti
Barilla ProteinPlus Thin Spaghetti
Barilla Veggie Spaghetti
Barilla White Fiber Spaghetti
Barilla White Fiber Thin Spaghetti
Barilla Whole Grain Angel Hair
Barilla Whole Grain Linguini
Barilla Whole Grain Spaghetti
Barilla Whole Grain Thin Spaghetti
Ezekiel 4:9 Sprouted Whole Grain Elbow Pasta

Ezekiel 4:9 Sprouted Whole Grain Fettuccine
Ezekiel 4:9 Sprouted Whole Grain Penne Pasta
Ezekiel 4:9 Sprouted Whole Grain Spaghetti
Racconto 8 Whole Grain Capellini
Racconto 8 Whole Grain Spaghetti
Ronzoni Healthy Harvest Ancient Grains Penne
Ronzoni Healthy Harvest Ancient Grains Thin Spaghetti
Ronzoni Healthy Harvest Lasagna
Ronzoni Healthy Harvest Linguini
Ronzoni Healthy Harvest Penne
Ronzoni Healthy Harvest Rotini
Sam Mills Pasta d'oro Corn Pasta

PASTA SAUCE

Every tomato sauce has sugar, thanks to the natural sugars in the tomatoes—but ones with added sugars can have 10 grams or more! The following popular brands have fewer than 6 grams of all-natural sugars.

Classico Riserva Eggplant & Artichoke
Classico Riserva Roasted Garlic
Classico Riserva Triple Olive Puttanesca
Classico Riserva Tomato Marinara
De Cecco Pesto alla Genovese
De Cecco Ragù alla Bolognese
De Cecco Sugo al basilico
De Cecco Sugo al pomodoro
De Cecco Sugo alla Napoletana
De Cecco Sugo alla Siciliana
De Cecco Sugo all'Arrabbiata
De Cecco Sugo alle olive
De Cecco Sugo delizie di verdure
Dell'Amore Original Recipe
Dell'Amore Romana
Dell'Amore Spicy Recipe
Dell'Amore Sweet Basil and Garlic
Hunt's Pasta Sauce No Added Sugar
Ragu Old World Style No Sugar Added Tomato Basil Sauce

Rao's Arrabbiata Sauce

Rao's Artichoke Sauce

Rao's 4 Cheese Sauce

Rao's Garden Vegetable Sauce

Rao's Homemade Marinara Sauce

Rao's Puttanesca Sauce

Rao's Roasted Eggplant Sauce

Rao's Roasted Garlic Sauce

Rao's Sensitive Formula Marinara

Rao's Tomato Basil Sauce

Rao's Vodka Sauce

OILS

Oils are sugar-free naturally, and the list below includes
the healthiest.

Almond Oil

Apricot kernel Oil

Babassu Oil

Canola Oil

Coconut Oil

Corn Oil

Cottonseed Oil

Extra-Virgin Olive Oil

Flaxseed Oil

Grapeseed Oil

Hazelnut Oil

Peanut Oil

Poppy Seed Oil

Safflower Oil

Sesame Oil

Sunflower Oil

Teaseed Oil

Walnut Oil

SOUPS

Alphabet or not, your soup spells S-U-G-A-R, since most major
brands include it as an ingredient. Not these.

Amy's Organic Black Bean Vegetable Soup

Amy's Organic Hearty Minestrone with Vegetables

Amy's Organic Lentil Soup

Amy's Organic Lentil Vegetable Soup

Amy's Organic Light in Sodium Lentil Vegetable Soup

Amy's Organic Mushroom Bisque with Porcini

Amy's Organic Quinoa, Kale & Red Lentil Soup

Amy's Organic Split Pea Soup

Amy's Organic Summer Corn & Vegetable Soup

Amy's Organic Vegan Chunky Tomato Bisque

Amy's Organic Vegetable Barley Soup

Campbell's Healthy Request Mexican-Style Chicken Tortilla

Campbell's Ready to Serve Low Sodium Chicken Broth

Campbell's Ready to Serve Low Sodium Chicken with Noodles Soup

Campbell's Ready to Serve Low Sodium Cream of Mushroom

BEANS AND LEGUMES

A tremendous source of protein, beans are best bought dry or low-sodium in cans.

Azuki Bean	Lentil
Black-Eyed Pea	Mung Bean
Black Bean	Navy Beans
Cannellini Beans	Pinto Beans
Chickpea/Garbanzo Bean	Soybean
Fava Bean	Tempeh
Great Northern Beans	Tiger Nuts
Kidney Beans	Tofu

NUTS

Obviously no sugar, buy a variety that have no added salt, for the heart-healthiest choice.

Almond	Peanut
Brazil Nut	Pecan
Cashew	Pine Nut
Hazelnut	Pistachio
Macadamia Nut	Walnut

SEEDS

The perfect topping for your plain yogurt, these also provide necessary fiber.

Chia	Sesame
Flax	Sunflower
Hemp	Tahini
Pumpkin	

BARS

Most nutrition and protein bars belong behind bars: They're filled with sugar and artificial sweeteners. But check out any flavors of the below:

Larabars

Manbake

RxBar

CRACKERS

After scouring the cracker aisle, I'm cracking up: Only one major brand is sugar free, Triscuit!

Blue Diamond Almond Nut Thins

Triscuit Garden Herb

Triscuit Hint of Salt

Triscuit Minis

Triscuit Original

Triscuit Reduced Fat

Triscuit Rye with Caraway Seeds

Triscuit Thin Crisps Originals

Note: Cheez-It Originals are also sugar-free, but because of their high sodium count, I don't recommend you eat them.

CHIPS

They're called junk food for a reason: Some chips have more sugar than cookies! In fact, almost every flavored chip has added sugars, even the simple salt-and-pepper flavor. But these don't:

Potato Chips

Food Should Taste Good Original Sweet Potato Chips

Good Health Kettle Chips Avocado Oil Sea Salt

Good Health Potato Popper Crisps Sea Salt

Grandma Utz's Regular Handcooked Potato Chips

Herr's Lightly Salted Potato Chips

Herr's Potato Chips Crisp 'n Tasty

Herr's Potato Chips Kettle Cooked
Kettle Brand Baked Olive Oil
Lay's Classic Potato Chips
Lay's Deli Style Original Potato Chips
Lay's Kettle Cooked Original
Lay's Kettle Cooked 40% Less Fat Original
Lay's Kettle Cooked Lattice Cut Sea Salt
Lay's Wavy Lightly Salted
Lay's Wavy Original
Ruffles Original
Ruffles Reduced Fat
Tyrell's Lightly Sea Salted
Tyrell's Veg Chips
Utz Kettle Classics 40% Reduced Fat
Utz Kettle Classics Gourmet Cut
Utz Kettle Classics Original
Utz No Salt Added Original Potato Chips
Utz Original Potato Chips
Utz Reduced Fat Original Potato Chips
Utz Reduced Fat Ripples Original Potato Chips
Utz Ripples Original Potato Chips
Utz Wavy Original Potato Chips
Wise Potato Chips Kettle Cooked Original
Wise Potato Chips Kettle Cooked Original 40% Reduced Fat
Wise Potato Chips Lightly Salted
Wise Potato Chips Original
Wise Potato Chips Ridgies All Natural
Wise Potato Chips Salt & Vinegar
Wise Potato Chips Unsalted

Corn Chips

Dipsy Doodles Original
Fritos Original
Fritos Scoops
Wise Original Flavor Corn Chips

Tortilla Chips

Garden of Eatin' Baked Blue Chips
Garden of Eatin' Baked Yellow Chips
Garden of Eatin' Black Bean
Garden of Eatin' Black Bean Chili
Garden of Eatin' Blue Corn Tortilla Chips
Garden of Eatin' Blue Corn Tortilla Chips Unsalted
Garden of Eatin' Little Soy Blues
Garden of Eatin' Mini White Corn Tortilla Rounds
Garden of Eatin' Mini White Strips
Garden of Eatin' Mini Yellow Rounds
Garden of Eatin' Pico de Gallo
Garden of Eatin' Red Corn Tortilla Chips
Garden of Eatin' Red Hot Blues
Garden of Eatin' Sesame Blues
Garden of Eatin' Sunny Blues
Garden of Eatin' Veggie Chips
Garden of Eatin' White Chips
Garden of Eatin' Yellow Chips
Herr's Bite Size Tortilla Chips
Herr's Tortilla Chips Restaurant Style
Snyder's of Hanover Dippin' Strips Tortilla Strips
Snyder's of Hanover Restaurant Style Tortilla Chips
Snyder's of Hanover White Corn Tortilla Chips
Tostitos Bite Size
Tostitos Cantina Thin & Crispy
Tostitos Cantina Traditional
Tostitos Crispy Rounds
Tostitos Original Restaurant Style
Tostitos Rolls
Tostitos Scoops
Way Better Black Bean
Way Better Blue Corn
Way Better Ginger Sweet Potato
Way Better Multi-Grain
Way Better No Salt Naked Blues
Wise White Restaurant Style Tortillas

Veggie or Legume-Based Chips
Good Health Veggie Chips Sea Salt
Good Health Veggie Straws Sea Salt
Plentils Light Sea Salt
Simply 7 Lentil Chips Sea Salt

Pretzels
Snyder's of Hanover Rods
Snyder's of Hanover Sourdough Hard Pretzels
Snyder's of Hanover Sourdough Nibblers

Other brands: Kettle Chips

POPCORN
Although many microwavable brands contain zero sugar,
I can't in good conscience recommend any here. Many major brands
like Jolly Time and Jiffy Pop not only contain heart-harming trans
fats but also line their bags with perfluorooctanoic acid (PFOA),
the same toxic stuff found in Teflon pots and pans. My preference:
Air pop kernels or make your own microwavable popcorn for a
low-calorie snack. Just add your favorite popping kernels to a small
paper lunch bag, and fold the top down a few times. Then zap it in
the microwave until you hear only a few pops every five seconds.

Or, enjoy these store-bought bagged brands:

Boom Chicka Pop Sea Salt
Boom Chicka Pop White Cheddar
Go Lite Himalayan Salt
Good Health Half Naked Hint of Olive Oil
Good Health Half Naked Organic Sea Salt
Good Health Half Naked Wild Buffalo Blue
SkinnyPop Jalapeño
SkinnyPop Original
SkinnyPop Sea Salt & Pepper
SkinnyPop White Cheddar
Smartfood Delight Sea Salt

DIPS AND SPREADS

You've heard of the "middle-age spread," and you'll get one if you eat dips loaded with added sugars. Fortunately, I found these delicious sugar-free options, so you can be the life of the party—and live a longer life.

Salsa

Amy's Salsa Mild, Medium, and Black Bean & Corn
Snyder's of Hanover Chunky Salsa Mild and Medium
Tostitos Chunky Salsa Mild, Medium, and Hot
Wise Salsa Mild and Medium

Guacamole

Wholly Guacamole—all varieties

Hummus

Athenos Artichoke Garlic Hummus
Athenos Black Olive Hummus
Athenos Greek Style Hummus
Athenos Original Hummus
Athenos Roasted Garlic Hummus
Athenos Roasted Red Pepper Hummus
Athenos Spicy Three Pepper Hummus
Cedar's Classic Original Hummus
Cedar's Everything Hummus
Cedar's Garlic Lovers Hummus
Cedar's Roasted Red Pepper Hummus
Cedar's Sundried Tomato & Basil Hummus
Food Should Taste Good Black Bean Hummus
Food Should Taste Good Chickpea and Lemon Hummus
Food Should Taste Good Chickpea Hummus
Sabra Basil Pesto Hummus
Sabra Chipotle Hummus
Sabra Classic Hummus
Sabra Lemon Twist Hummus
Sabra Olive Tapenade Hummus
Sabra Roasted Garlic Hummus

Sabra Roasted Pine Nut Hummus
Sabra Rosemary with Sea Salt Hummus
Sabra Spinach and Artichoke Hummus
Sabra Supremely Spicy Hummus
Sabra Tuscan Herb Garden Hummus
Tribe Classic Hummus
Tribe Mediterranean Style Hummus
Tribe Roasted Garlic Hummus
Tribe Spicy Red Pepper Hummus
Tribe Swirl Salsa Hummus
Tribe Zesty Spice & Garlic Hummus

DRESSINGS

Although *Zero Sugar Diet* doesn't recommend artificial sweeteners, a touch in your dressing—like the Splenda in Walden Farms brands—is allowed. But all you really need to dress a salad is olive oil and balsamic vinegar.

Annie's Naturals Organic Oil and Vinegar
Walden Farms Asian
Walden Farms Bacon Ranch
Walden Farms Balsamic Vinaigrette
Walden Farms Bleu Cheese
Walden Farms Buttermilk Ranch
Walden Farms Caesar
Walden Farms Chipotle Ranch
Walden Farms Coleslaw
Walden Farms Creamy Bacon
Walden Farms Creamy Italian
Walden Farms French
Walden Farms Honey Balsamic Vinaigrette
Walden Farms Honey Dijon
Walden Farms Italian
Walden Farms Italian Sun Dried Tomato
Walden Farms Jersey Sweet Onion
Walden Farms Pear & White Balsamic Vinaigrette
Walden Farms Raspberry Vinaigrette

Walden Farms Russian
Walden Farms Sesame Ginger
Walden Farms Super Fruits Balsamic Vinaigrette
Walden Farms Thousand Island
Walden Farms Zesty Italian

BAKING

Enjoy all of the below—but surprise, there's no "sugar"
on the list.

Baker's yeast
Baking chocolate, unsweetened, liquid
Baking powder
Baking soda
Corn bran, crude
Cornstarch
Cream of tartar
Gelatin, unsweetened
Lard

ICE CREAMS AND FROZEN TREATS

Cookies, Candy Bars

There is no such thing as sugar-free ice cream, because ice
cream is made with sugar! Same goes for cookies and candy bars.
For the first fourteen days of *Zero Sugar Diet*, you won't lay a finger
on a Butterfinger.

Beverages

Coffee, tea, and sparkling waters are all allowed on *The Zero
Sugar Diet*, provided you don't load them up with sugar. And I even
found some wines with less than 1 gram of sugar per 5-ounce
serving! Sip off the pounds with:

Plant-based Milks

Blue Diamond Unsweetened
Pacific Unsweetened
Silk Unsweetened
SoDelicious Unsweetened

Bottled Teas

Honest Tea Just Unsweetened
Inko's White Tea Unsweetened
Pure Leaf Unsweetened
Tejava Unsweetened

Wines

Cabernet Sauvignon
Chardonnay
Italian Pinot Grigio
Pinot Noir
Sauvignon Blanc

For 1,000+ more no-sugar-added products and Zero Sugar–approved restaurant dishes, go to **thezerosugardiet.com**!

ACKNOWLEDGMENTS

This book would not have been possible without the support, guidance, and hard work of the following:

The many test panelists who tried *Zero Sugar Diet* and saw amazing results—and the millions of fans at eatthis.com.

Marnie Cochran, a brilliant editor with a golden gut.

Gina Centrello, Kara Welsh, Bill Takes, Kim Hovey, Jennifer Hershey, Joe Perez, Nina Shield, Susan Corcoran, Theresa Zoro, Cindy Murray, Scott Shannon, Matt Schwartz, Toby Ernst, and Quinne Rogers at Ballantine.

Stephen Perrine.

Michael Freidson, George Karabotsos, Jon Hammond, Sean Bumgarner, Jeff Csatari, Christie Griffin, John Phalen, Dana Smith, Daniel Cohen, Daniel McCarter, Olivia Tarantino, Charlene Lutz, and the entire team at Galvanized Media.

Ben Sherwood, Barbara Fedida, Patty Neger, and the teams at *Good Morning America* and ABC News.

Jennifer Rudolph Walsh, Jon Rosen, Andy McNicol, and the amazing talents at WME.

Larry Shire, Eric Sacks, and Jonathan Erlich, who provide invaluable counsel.

Nutritionist Carly Smolnik.

Mehmet Oz, David Pecker, Steve Lacy, Strauss Zelnick, Dan Abrams, Dr. Jennifer Ashton, Michele Promaulayko, and the many friends and colleagues who continue to inspire me with their wisdom and acumen.

And the best family a man could ever hope for.

INDEX

ABOUT THE AUTHORS

DAVID ZINCZENKO is the *New York Times* bestselling author of *Zero Belly Diet, Zero Belly Cookbook,* and *Zero Belly Smoothies,* the co-author of the Eat This, Not That! franchise (which has sold more than eight million copies worldwide), and the Abs Diet books. Currently the editorial director at *Men's Fitness,* he is the award-winning former editor in chief of *Men's Health* and editorial director of *Women's Health, Prevention,* and *Best Life* magazines. Zinczenko is also the nutrition and wellness editor at ABC News and the CEO of the media company Galvanized, where he runs eatthis.com and bestlifeonline.com. He lives in New York City.

thezerosugardiet.com
Facebook.com/thezerosugardiet
@zerosugardiet

To inquire about booking David Zinczenko for a speaking engagement, please contact the Penguin Random House Speakers Bureau at speakers@penguinrandomhouse.com.

STEPHEN PERRINE is the author of *The Men's Health Diet* and *The New American Diet.* The former publisher of Rodale Books and editor in chief of *Best Life,* he lives in New York City.